Communicable disease control in emergencies

A field manual

Edited by M.A. Connolly

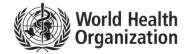

**World Health
Organization**

WHO Library Cataloguing-in-Publication Data

Communicable disease control in emergencies: a field manual edited by
M. A. Connolly.

    1. Communicable disease control–methods 2. Emergencies 3. Disease
outbreak, prevention and control 4. Manuals I. Connolly, Máire A.

ISBN 92 4 154616 6   (NLM Classification: WA 110)

WHO/CDS/2005.27

Layout: CME/B. Duret, France – Photo credits: top left & bottom: Unicef / middle: PAHO / top right: WHO–Gayer

CONTENTS

4 OUTBREAK CONTROL

5 DISEASE PREVENTION AND CONTROL

ANNEXES

ACKNOWLEDGEMENTS

Edited by Máire Connolly, WHO/CDS.

Rick Brennan (IRC), Philippe Calain (WHO/CDS), Michelle Gayer (WHO/CDS), Tim Healing (Merlin), Myriam Henkens (MSF), Jean Long (Trinity College, Dublin), Serge Male (UNHCR), Pamela Mbabazi (WHO/CDS), Agostino Paganini (UNICEF), Jean Rigal (MSF), Mike Ryan (WHO/EPR), Peter Salama (CDC), Paul Spiegel (CDC), Mike Toole (Macfarlane Burnet Centre for Medical Research and Public Health) and Ron Waldman (Mailman School of Public Health, Columbia University) contributed extensively to the development of this manual.

The following people contributed to the development and review of this document and their input is gratefully acknowledged:

Samira Aboubaker (WHO/CAH), Nathalie Agata (WHO/Ethiopia), Roberta Andraghetti (WHO/EPR), Ray Arthur (WHO/EPR), O. Babu-Swai (UNHCR, Kenya), Andrew Ball (WHO/HIV), Claudio Beltramello (WHO/CPE), Sylvie Briand (WHO/NTD), Nan Buzard (Sphere Project), Claire-Lise Chaignat (WHO/NTD), Claire Chauvin (WHO/IVB), Denis Coulombier (WHO/EPR), Charles Delacollette (WHO/RBM), Mike Deppner (UNHCR, Uganda), Philippe Desjeux (WHO/CPE), Hans Everts (WHO/IVB), Albis Francesco Gabrielli (WHO/CPE), Bernardus Ganter (WHO/EURO), Antonio Gerbase (WHO/HIV), Robin Gray (WHO/EDM), Tom Grein (WHO/EPR), Malgosia Grzemska (WHO/STB), Pierre Guillet (WHO/NTD), Zoheir Hallaj (WHO/EMRO), Max Hardiman (WHO/EPR), Christopher Haskew (WHO/CPE), Mary Healy (Trocaire, Ireland), Ana Maria Henao-Restrepo (WHO/IVB), Brad Hersh (WHO/IVB), David Heymann (WHO/CDS), Gottfried Hirnschall (WHO/HIV), Jose Hueb (WHO/PHE), Yvan Hutin (WHO/IVB), Jean Jannin (WHO/NTD),

Vijay Kumar (WHO/SEARO), Joël Lagoutte (ICRC, Geneva), Daniel Lavanchy (WHO/EPR), Dominique Legros (Epicentre), Alessandro Loretti (WHO/HAC), Paul Lusamba-Dikassa (WHO/AFRO), Chris Maher (WHO/Polio), Frédérique Marodon (WHO/CPE), Adelheid Marschang (IFRC), Zahra Mirghani (UNHCR), Lulu Muhe (WHO/CAH), Mike Nathan (WHO/NTD), Maria Neira (WHO/CPE), Hitoshi Oshitani (WHO/WPRO), Brian Pazvakavambwa (WHO/HIV), William Perea (WHO/EPR), Pierre Perrin (ICRC), Aafje Rietveld (WHO/RBM), Guénaël Rodier (WHO/CSR), Cathy Roth (WHO/EPR), Maria Santamaria (WHO/CSR), Akihiro Seita (WHO/EMRO), Khalid Shibib (WHO/HAC), Eigil Sorensen (WHO/DPRKorea), John Tabayi (UNHCR, Ethiopia), Nadia Teleb (WHO/EMRO), Jan Theunissen (WHO/EURO), Michel Thuriaux (WHO/CSR), A. Tijtsma (UNHCR), Kaat Vandemacle (WHO/EPR), Claude de Ville de Goyet (WHO/ PAHO), Zita Weise Prinzo (WHO/NHD), Brad Woodruff (CDC), Nevio Zagaria (WHO/CPE).

WHO would like to thank the Government of Ireland for its support in the development of this manual.

INTRODUCTION

This manual is intended to help health professionals and public health coordinators working in emergency situations prevent, detect and control the major communicable diseases encountered by affected populations. Emergencies include complex emergencies and natural disasters (e.g. floods and earthquakes). The term "complex emergencies" has been coined to describe "situations of war or civil strife affecting large civilian populations with food shortages and population displacement, resulting in excess mortality and morbidity".

In this manual, the generic term "emergencies" will be used to encompass all situations in which large populations are in need of urgent humanitarian relief. Following an emergency, the affected population is often displaced and temporarily resettled. They may be placed in camps or become dispersed among the local population (either in towns or in rural communities). People who are displaced across national borders are termed refugees whereas those who have been displaced within their country are called "internally displaced persons" (IDPs). Resettlement in camps may entail high population densities, inadequate shelter, poor water supplies and sanitation, and a lack of even basic health care. In these situations, there is an increased threat of communicable disease and a high risk of epidemics.

Communicable diseases are a major cause of mortality and morbidity in emergencies, and particularly in complex emergencies, where collapsing health services and disease control programmes, poor access to health care, malnutrition, interrupted supplies and logistics, and poor coordination among the various agencies providing health care often coexist. The main causes of morbidity and mortality in emergencies are diarrhoeal diseases, acute respiratory infections, measles and, in areas where it is endemic, malaria. Other communicable diseases, such as epidemic meningococcal disease, tuberculosis, relapsing fever and typhus, have also caused large epidemics among emergency-affected populations. Malnutrition and trauma are the two main additional causes of illness and death.

Ensuring adequate shelter, water, sanitation and food and providing basic health care are the most effective means of protecting the health of those affected by emergencies. A systematic approach to the control of communicable diseases is a key component of humanitarian response, and is crucial to protect the health of affected populations. This requires co-operation among agencies working at local, national and international levels, and collaboration among all sectors involved in the emergency response – health, food and nutrition, shelter, water and sanitation.

This field manual is the result of collaboration among a number of WHO departments and several external partner agencies in reviewing existing guidelines on communicable disease control and adapting them to emergency situations. This manual deals with the fundamental principles of communicable disease control in emergencies, which are:

- **RAPID ASSESSMENT**: identify the communicable disease threats faced by the emergency-affected population, including those with epidemic potential, and define the health status of the population, by conducting a rapid assessment;

- **PREVENTION:** prevent communicable disease by maintaining a healthy physical environment and good general living conditions;

- **SURVEILLANCE:** set up or strengthen disease surveillance system with an early warning mechanism to ensure the early reporting of cases, to monitor disease trends, and to facilitate prompt detection and response to outbreaks;

- **OUTBREAK CONTROL:** ensure outbreaks are rapidly detected and controlled through adequate preparedness (i.e. stockpiles, standard treatment protocols and staff training) and rapid response (i.e. confirmation, investigation and implementation of control measures); and

- **DISEASE MANAGEMENT:** diagnose and treat cases promptly with trained staff using effective treatment and standard protocols at all health facilities.

It is hoped that this manual, by setting standards for communicable disease control in emergencies, will promote effective, coordinated action towards the prevention and control of communicable diseases in emergencies. Where appropriate, the manual provides suggestions for further reading, with references to relevant background material, guidelines and reviews. Finally, whilst shelter, food, water and sanitation sectors are covered, this manual specifically aims to provide detail on health issues.

Steps in ensuring communicable disease control in emergencies

---

Conduct rapid health assessment
- Identify main disease threats, including potential epidemic diseases
- Obtain data on the host country, on the country of origin of displaced persons and on the areas through which they may have passed
- Identify priority public health interventions
- Identify the lead health agency
- Establish health coordination mechanisms

Prevent communicable diseases
- Select and plan sites
- Ensure adequate water and sanitation facilities
- Ensure availability of food
- Control vectors
- Implement vaccination campaigns (e.g. measles)
- Provide essential clinical services
- Provide basic laboratory facilities

Set up surveillance/early warning system
- Detect outbreaks early
- Report diseases of epidemic potential immediately
- Monitor disease trends

Control outbreaks

Preparation	– outbreak response team
	– stockpiles
	– laboratory support
	– standard treatment protocols
Detection	– surveillance/early warning system
Confirmation	– laboratory tests
Response	– investigation
	– control measures
Evaluation	

1. RAPID ASSESSMENT

A rapid health assessment must be conducted as soon as possible after an emergency, ideally within one week. The aim is to identify the main communicable disease threats, outline the public health needs and plan priority interventions. The duration of a rapid assessment depends on the size and geographical distribution of the population affected, the security situation, the conditions of access, transport and logistics, the human resources available and the methods used. It should be completed within one week, depending on the extent of the emergency.

A more thorough assessment, with detailed qualitative and quantitative data and intervention plans, should be completed as soon as possible after the rapid assessment. The assessment must be undertaken by well-qualified and experienced epidemiologists. The key activities involved in a rapid assessment are outlined in Table 1.1.

Table 1.1   **Key activities in rapid assessment**

1. Planning the mission
Composition of the health assessment team
Collection of background geopolitical data
Collection of background health data on host country and country of origin

2. Field visit
Data: demography, environment, health data, resource needs
Methods: aerial inspection; direct observation; interviews with agencies, the ministry of health and local authorities; collection of health data from medical facilities; rapid estimation of population size by mapping, review of records and rapid surveys

3. Analysis
Demographic pyramids
Priority health interventions
Identification of high-risk groups

4. Report writing

5. Dissemination

1.1   Objectives

The objectives of a rapid assessment are:
- to assess the extent of the emergency and the communicable disease threat to the population;
- to define the type and size of interventions and priority activities;
- to plan the implementation of these activities;
- to pass information to the international community, donors and the media in order to mobilize human and financial resources.

1.2 Composition of the team

The rapid health assessment team should consist of:
- a public health expert/epidemiologist,
- a nutritionist,
- a logistician/administrative officer,
- a water and sanitation/environmental health specialist.

One member must be designated as team leader.

The tasks of the team during this initial phase are to:
- prepare a rapid health assessment checklist,
- prepare a timetable of assessment,
- assign tasks,
- obtain necessary equipment (e.g. computers, scales, laboratory supplies),
- organize visas, transport, vehicles, fuel,
- set up a communication system,
- inform the local authorities,
- inform potential donors and key decision-makers.

1.3 Methods of data collection

The collection of data in an emergency may not proceed in a step-by-step manner, but the plan for data collection and analysis must be systematic.

The four main methods of collecting data are:
- review of existing information,
- visual inspection of the affected area,
- interviews with key informants,
- rapid surveys.

1.3.1 Review of existing information

A review should be undertaken of baseline health and other information available at national and regional levels, from government, international and nongovernmental sources, concerning:
- the geographical and environmental characteristics of the country and affected area (e.g. national, subnational and district maps showing administrative and political divisions of the affected area, settlements, water sources, main transport routes and health facilities);
- the size, composition and prior health and nutritional condition of the emergency-affected population;
- the health services and programmes functioning before and during the emergency;

- the resources already allocated, obtained or requested for the emergency response operation;
- the security situation.

1.3.2   Visual inspection of the affected area

Where travel is by air, useful observations of the affected area can be made before landing. An initial walk or drive through the area may allow for a first rough idea of the adequacy of shelter, food availability, environmental factors such as drainage and risks of vector breeding, and the general status of the population.

During the initial visual inspection, the area should be mapped, even if only crudely. The resulting maps should indicate the affected area, the distribution of the population and the location of resources (medical facilities, water sources, food distribution points, temporary shelters, etc.).

Mapping also allows the estimation of population data, through the calculation of the total surface area of the camp and of sections of the camps. The method is based on the making of a map of the camp, with its different sections. By using random sampling of several known surface areas one may count the number of persons living in these zones and establish the average population per area. One can calculate the total population of the camp by extrapolating the average population per square into the total surface area of the site (see example).

1.3.3   Interviews with key informants

Interviews must be conducted with key personnel in the area and with the affected population, and must include people from all sectors of the population involved:

- clan, village and community leaders,
- area administrators or other governmental officials,
- health workers, including traditional birth attendants, healers, etc.,
- personnel from local and international emergency response organizations, including United Nations organizations,
- individuals in the affected population.

Community organizational structures, normal dietary practices, cultural practices relating to water and hygiene, and preferences for health care should all be recorded.

1.3.4   Rapid surveys

Rapid surveys take time and should be reserved for essential data not available from other sources. They may be used to determine the sex and age distribution of the population, the average family size, the number of people in vulnerable groups, recent mortality rates (retrospective mortality study), the main causes of mortality and morbidity, current nutritional status, vaccination coverage, and the use of formal and informal health services. Techniques are rather well codified, and are based on validated sampling and analysis methods in order to provide quantitative estimates of the situation with reasonable accuracy and within acceptable delays. This is essential (a) to guide emergency decisions on where and when resources should be allocated, and (b) as a baseline for monitoring interventions. Surveys and sampling methods are outlined below. Sample household survey and rapid assessment forms are included in Annex 2.

1.4   Survey and sampling methods

1.4.1   Introduction

The first priority when entering an emergency area for the first time is to undertake a needs assessment so as to ensure an effective use of limited resources. Inadequate or incomplete assessments can lead to inappropriate responses and waste of scarce resources, and personnel may be needlessly endangered.

While most assessments will be a straightforward data collection exercise, a structured and statistically analysable survey may be needed to answer a particular question. It is equally important to undertake re-surveys at intervals, so as to keep abreast of a changing situation. This forms an important part of ongoing surveillance. The use of a standard method throughout means that the results of different surveys/assessments can be compared directly. Any changes quickly become apparent. The use of such methods makes it easier to monitor the response and determine its effectiveness.

If possible, advice should be taken from a biometrician before formal surveys are undertaken, as it is important to structure the survey so as to get representative and easily analysable results.

When possible use EpiInfo and EpiData for all aspects of data entry and handling.

It is important to understand that there may be security implications of undertaking surveys and assessments in chaotic, unstable situations. Local people may view questionnaires with suspicion: they may not understand the idea of the survey and feel that (for example) they are being earmarked for deportation. Some form of advance publicity may be necessary, but should be undertaken carefully so as not to bias any samples. The survey/assessment may need to be undertaken rapidly if the situation is dangerous.

In addition to the rapid needs assessment, good epidemiological surveillance should be put in place as soon as possible.

Rapid needs assessment should not be viewed in isolation but as one aspect of surveillance in emergency situations.

Attempts should also be made to:

- secure data from other sources (e.g. clinic data, local authorities, other nongovernmental organizations, community leaders, etc.);
- ensure that there is ongoing surveillance, possibly using sentinel surveillance points, repeat surveys;
- regularly analyse existing health clinic data, etc.

1.4.2   Surveys

Although the ideal would be to measure the whole of a population, this is rarely possible (it may occasionally be so in a small refugee camp). In practice a sample must be taken. The sample should be representative of the population, but a balance must be struck between the ideal and the attainable. In emergencies there is always a trade-off between rapidity and accuracy.

The size of the sample must be adequate to accomplish what is required, but not wasteful. In an emergency the size of a sample may be governed by factors other than immediate statistical requirements (e.g. accessibility, staff availability, security, etc.).

There are several essential steps to be followed in any survey:

1. Defining the aims clearly

This is the crucial first step, as all other aspects of the survey stem from this. Most surveys have multiple aims. The key reasons for an agency to undertake a survey are to ensure that the appropriate aid is sent to those who need it in the acute phase of the emergency, and to have a baseline from which to monitor the effect.

It is important not to try to collect too many items of data in one survey. Define what you need to know, not what you would like to know. Consider cost, speed, available resources and security.

2. Selecting the site

You need to decide which area you want to have information about. This could be, for example, a province, a city, the area where an agency is active or a damaged area of a city (if a large part was untouched). The area selected should be clearly defined, together with the reasons for its selection. A suitable control area may need to be selected. If you are working in a devastated area, an untouched area might be needed at the same time for comparison.

3. Defining the basic sampling unit

In random sampling methods the basic sampling unit is usually individuals, whereas in a cluster survey it is usually occupied households. Whatever definition is chosen, it should be stated in the report.

4. Sample size

The size of the sample should ideally be based on how reliable the final estimates must be. A sample must represent the population as a whole. Each individual should have an equal chance of being sampled, and the selection of an individual should be independent of the selection of any other.

➜ *For calculating the sample size for a proportion:*

The following items determine the size of the sample needed.

✔ *The confidence level and precision required*

The use of a sample means that only an estimate of the results from the whole population is obtained. Subsequent samples are likely to give different values, but provided the samples have been selected correctly there will be little variation between them. The actual population value will lie in a range around the observed value(s). The confidence interval is the upper and lower limits of this range (e.g. result = 12% ± 2%; the confidence interval is 10–14%). The size of the confidence interval is related to the error risk and the sample size. The greater the precision required, the larger the sample must be.

✔ *The variability of the characteristics being measured in the study population*

If this is unknown you must assume maximum variability.

✔ *The size of the population under study*

Usually what is required is to find out what proportion of a population has some characteristic. When this type of information is sought, sample size is determined using the following formula:

$$n = \frac{t^2 \times p \times q}{d^2}$$

where: n = first estimate of sample size

t = confidence (for 95% use 1.96)

d = precision (usually 0.05 or 0.10)

p = proportion of the target population with the characteristics being measured (if proportion is unknown, let p = 0.5)

$q = 1 - p$

Once n is calculated, compare it with the size of the target population (N). If n is known (or strongly suspected) to be less than 10% of N, then use n as the final sample size. If n >10% N, then use the following correction formula to recalculate the final sample size (n_f). (If the sample size is >10% of the population a smaller sample can be used.)

$$n_f = \frac{n}{1 - n/N}$$

Once n_f has been determined, you need to decide whether it is possible to achieve that sample size under the circumstances of the mission. If not, a smaller sample size may have to be accepted with the caveat that this will reduce precision.

As an example, we have a population where the expected disease rate is 12%. We need to measure the prevalence with a precision of 2%. The sample size required is:

$$n = \frac{1.96^2 \times 0.12 \times 0.88}{0.02^2} = 1014$$

However, the population size is known to be 6000 and this sample size is therefore >10% of the population size.

$$\text{revised } n = \frac{1014}{1 - 1014/6000} = 867$$

To assist you, some sample sizes with an error risk of 5% are given in Table 1.2. (NB. These are not revised sample sizes.)

Table 1.2   **Sample size according to expected prevalence in a random or systematic sample with an error risk of 5%**

Prevalence	Precision				
	1%	2%	3%	4%	5%
5%	1825	456	203	–	–
6%	2167	542	241	135	–
7%	2501	625	278	156	100
8%	2827	707	314	177	113
9%	3146	787	350	197	126
10%	3457	864	384	216	138
11%	3761	940	418	235	150
12%	4057	1014	451	254	162
13%	4345	1086	483	272	174
14%	4625	1156	514	289	185
15%	4898	1225	544	306	196
16%	5163	1291	574	323	207
17%	5420	1355	602	339	217
18%	5670	1418	630	354	227
19%	5912	1478	657	370	236
20%	6147	1537	683	384	246
30%	8067	2017	896	504	323
40%	9220	2305	1024	576	369
50%	9604	2401	1067	600	384

➜ *For calculating the sample size for a mean, for example the population mean:*

When sample data is collected and the sample mean χ is calculated, that sample mean is typically different from the true population mean μ. This difference between the sample and population means can be thought of as an error. The margin of error E is the maximum difference between the observed sample mean χ and the true value of the population mean μ:

$$E = z_{\alpha/2} \times \frac{\sigma}{\sqrt{n}}$$

where: $z_{\alpha/2}$ is the "critical value", the positive value z that is at the vertical boundary for the area of $\alpha/2$ in the right tail of the standard normal distribution

σ is the population standard deviation

n is the sample size

Rearranging this formula, the sample size necessary can be calculated to give results accurate to a specified confidence interval and margin of error.

$$n = \left[\frac{z_{\alpha/2} \times \sigma}{E} \right]^2$$

This formula is used when you know σ and want to determine the sample size necessary to establish the mean value μ, with a confidence of $(1 - \alpha)$, within $\pm E$ of error. This formula can still be used if the population standard deviation σ is unknown and you have a small sample size. Although it is unlikely that the standard deviation σ is known when the population mean is not known, σ may be determined from a similar process or from a pilot test/simulation.

5. The interview/questionnaire

Only collect information that will be used. Keep questions simple and unambiguous with yes/no answers as often as possible. Keep as short as possible to save time. Teams should be well trained and not allowed to introduce personal bias into the sampling. The people chosen should be acceptable and non-intimidating to the general population.

You may wish to build checks into the questionnaire. For example, two questions may be included at different places in the questionnaire that are differently worded but whose answers are the same in whole or in part. If very different answers are received, the veracity of the respondent may be questionable.

It may be necessary to select times of day for interviews when people are likely to be available.

1.4.3　Sampling methods

The following methods are discussed:

1. Census
2. Simple random sampling
3. Systematic sampling
4. Stratified sampling
5. Cluster sampling

1. Census

A census involves determining the size of a population and (often) obtaining other data at the same time. All the individuals (or at least representatives of all individuals, such as heads of families) need to be interviewed. This may be useful in well-defined populations such as refugee camps but can be extremely time consuming. Registration of refugees is notoriously unreliable, especially where food is concerned. The situation in acute emergencies is often chaotic and dynamic. Previous census data are often meaningless owing to massive population movements. Census data may be required to determine parameters such as rates of infection in well-defined populations (such as refugee camps), but such data can usually be obtained from the agency running the camp.

2. Simple random sampling

Random sampling is the only way of meeting the two criteria: that each individual should have an equal chance of being sampled, and the selection of an individual should be independent of the selection of any other. The individuals to be questioned (the "sampling units") are selected purely by chance from a complete list of the entire population being studied. (For example, each individual can be given a number and then numbers selected from the total list by use of random number tables.)

This is a statistically reliable method but can be time consuming and requires an *accurate* list of the individuals in the area. Determining the appropriate size of the sample can be a problem. The list of individuals could come from refugee registers, census data, tax registers, electoral registers, etc. In a war with shifting populations such reliable data rarely exist and this limits the use of this method. It may be appropriate in refugee camps with good registration data. No control over the distribution of the sample is exercised, so some samples may be unrepresentative.

There are a number of specialized techniques, based on random sampling, that are designed to ensure representative samples.

Tables of random numbers can be generated by Excel in the following way:

– launch Excel

– enter the following formula in the top left corner cell of the table that you want to produce: =RAND()*100

– you can increase the range of values returned by the formula by adjusting the value 100 in the formula. If 100 is replaced by *n*, random numbers from 0 to (*n* – 1) will be produced.

– set the decimals to 0 by using the "Format" and "Cell" menu options, and "Number" and "Decimal places" tabs

– copy the cell containing the formula to the range of the table to be produced

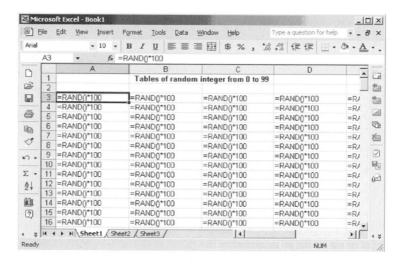

Tables of random numbers can be generated by Epi Info in the following way:

– run EPED from the EPI6 menu

– make a questionnaire file containing only one field: Number ######

– run ENTER and make a .REC file called RANDOM but do not enter any records

– press <F10> to return to the EPI6 menu

– run ANALYSIS from the EPI6 menu and READ RANDOM

– set up the random integers:

NUMBER = RAN(100)

GENERATE 1000

The integers will be placed in the file. You can now use the commands LIST NUMBER, FREQ NUMBER or LINE NUMBER to check the distribution. To print them for use, use ROUTE PRINTER followed by LIST NUMBER. If you want real numbers instead of integers, the RND(100) command will produce these.

3. Systematic sampling

This method is used when individuals or households (sampling units) can be ordered or listed in some manner. Rather than selecting all subjects randomly, a selection interval is determined (e.g. every fifth individual) a starting point on the list picked at random and every n^{th} person, household, etc. is selected (where n = the sampling interval) on the list. Good geographical distribution (according to population density) can be assured.

However, sampling units do not need to be listed in emergency situations as long as:

- the total number of units can be estimated,
- the enumerators can go through the area and pass in front of each sampling unit, selecting every x^{th} unit.

Systematic sampling allows better representativeness than simple random sampling (assuming there is no cyclic pattern in the distribution of sampling units and which would be extremely rare).

Example – Systematic sampling

Number of households: 6000

Sample size: 450 households

Sample interval: 6000/450 = 13 households

Information is collected every 13 households if the departure number is chosen at random between 1 and the sample interval.

If for example the departure number is 5 (thus the fifth household beginning at one extremity of the camp), then the selected households are numbers:

     5, then **18** (5+13); then **31** (18+13); then **44** (31+13), etc.

---

4. Stratified sampling

In this method the target population is divided into suitable, non-overlapping subpopulations (strata). Each stratum should be homogeneous within and heterogeneous between strata. A random sample is then selected within each stratum. Separate estimates can be obtained from each stratum, and an overall estimate obtained for the whole population defined by the strata. The value of this technique is that each stratum is accurately represented and overall sampling error is reduced.

5. Cluster sampling

One of the difficulties faced in most disasters is that the size of a population may not be known. The EPI (Extended Programme on Vaccination) cluster sampling method is often used to overcome this difficulty, as it is reliable, relatively cheap and rapid. It was originally developed to assess levels of smallpox coverage, and has been extended for use in other vaccination programmes. It is designed to produce representative samples even if the population size is unknown. Both qualitative and quantitative data can be collected. This method has been used in emergency situations.

Cluster sampling methods are also valuable when a population is geographically dispersed. The units sampled first are not members of the population but clusters (aggregates) of the population. The clusters are selected in such a fashion that they are representative of the population as a whole. For example, in a rural area a sample of villages may be selected and then some or all of the households included in the sample. A major advantage of this approach is that there is a saving of resources (reduced travelling, fewer staff) but the method lacks precision when compared to random sampling.

The EPI technique has been modified for use in nutritional surveys. A further development for the rapid assessment of health needs in disasters uses the technique to assess multiple aims, and consequently the basic sampling unit is no longer the individual but the household.

A variant of this method, which has been used in emergency situations, is the Modified two-stage cluster sampling method.

It is important to realize the limitations of this survey technique.

- The simple 30×7 "EPI" design is adequate for relatively frequent events (e.g. looking at vaccination status in the under-5s (when your sampling unit would be children under 5) but will not provide accurate estimates of relatively rare events such as mortality. To do this a much larger sample size would be needed.

- The technique does not meet the second criterion for representativeness, because the selection of an individual in a cluster is *not* independent of the selection of other individuals. Members of a cluster are likely to be similar. This is known as the "design effect" and may be especially serious with communicable diseases owing to their tendency to cluster close together. If questions about mortality and specific diseases are asked then great care should be taken not to draw too many firm conclusions from the results. Cluster sampling is more suited to questions related to, for example, access to health care, people currently ill, or need and availability of medication. The design effect can be countered to some degree by doubling the size of the sample required in random or systematic sampling. Design effect as such does not affect the point estimate calculated on the sample, but the precision (variance) only. The decrease in precision can be calculated during analysis by comparing the variance between clusters over the global variance.

The use of this technique in emergencies needs further rigorous evaluation, but in the mean time it seems to be the best method for data collection in urban areas that have been devastated by war or natural disaster.

The EPI method usually samples 30 clusters from the area of interest and then 7 subjects from adjacent households. (In principle the more clusters the better the randomness, but it should be balanced against time and cost.)

An example of cluster sampling is given below. The population of different sections in a settlement must be known. This method is divided into two stages as described below.

Stage 1: Selection of clusters

- Calculate cumulative population total (for example, population = 9300)

- Calculate the sampling interval

  For a cluster sampling survey, a sample of 30 clusters of 30 households is recommended (representing approximately 4000 to 5000 persons, of which 900 are children between 6 and 59 months)

  The desired sample size is, therefore, 30 clusters of 30 households = 900 households

  The sample interval for selecting the clusters is then calculated;

  e.g. **9300/30 − 310**

- Determine the first cluster by drawing, at random, a number between 1 and the sample interval (example in table − 170)

  The other clusters are then positioned in the cumulative list (170 + 310 = 480, etc.) and a number of clusters per section derived

Population per section	Cumulative total	Number of clusters per section	#
1 = 500	500	(170, 480)	2
2 = 2000	2500	(790, 1100, 1410, 1720, 2030, 2340)	6
3 = 1500	4000	(2650, 2960, 3270, 3580, 3890)	5
4 = 1000	5000	(4200, 4510, 4820)	3
5 = 1300	6300	(5130, 5440, 5750, 6060)	4
6 = 3000	9300	(6370, 6680, 6990, 7300, 7610, 7920, 8230, 8540, 8850, 9160)	10
Population total	9300		

Stage 2: Selection of individuals

• A direction is chosen at random from the centre of each section, and the number of households counted from the centre to the periphery in this direction.

• A number between 1 and the number of households counted is chosen at random. This number corresponds to the household that is the departure point for the selection of individuals in the cluster.

• In each cluster, households are selected by moving from one household to the nearest household, until the required cluster size is obtained (a target of 30 households per cluster is recommended).

• When children from 6 to 59 months are the target of the survey and there are several of these children in one household, one is chosen at random from each household.

If several clusters have been selected in one section, the same operation is repeated from the centre of the section.

Note: When possible, systematic sampling should be chosen by preference over cluster sampling. It is easier to carry out and, above all, is more rapid (one is able to obtain a precision of results equivalent to cluster sampling, but with a much smaller sample size).

1.5   Data to be collected

Data should be collected in the following areas:
• background health information,
• demography,
• mortality,
• morbidity,
• health services and infrastructure,
• food,
• nutritional status,
• water,
• sanitation,
• shelter and non-food items,
• environment,
• coordination.

1.5.1   Background health information

Background health information comprises:
• the main health and nutritional problems,
• coverage by public health programmes (e.g. vaccination coverage rates),

- the health care infrastructure, staff available and use of traditional medicine,
- the availability of health workers,
- important health beliefs and traditions,
- social organization.

When displaced populations are at the centre of the humanitarian emergency, similar data should be collected on their place of origin.

If possible, background information should be collected before the field mission is conducted, using as sources the Ministry of Health, WHO, international and nongovernmental organizations and WHO web sites.

In the field, data should be collected through interviews with community leaders, heads of households, health workers and individuals.

1.5.2   Demography

Demographic information comprises:
- total population size (displaced persons and host population);
- population under 5 years of age;
- ethnic composition and place of origin;
- sex ratio;
- the number of persons in the following high-risk groups: pregnant and lactating women, members of households headed by a woman, unaccompanied children, disabled and wounded people, and the elderly;
- the average size of a family/household;
- the number of arrivals and departures per week;
- the predicted number of future arrivals;
- activity patterns in the host (and possibly the displaced) populations that may affect the timing of surveys (e.g. when people go to collect water, to the fields, etc.).

The following sources can be used for retrieving demographic data:
- mapping;
- aerial or satellite pictures;
- census data;
- records maintained by camp administrators, local government officials, United Nations organizations, religious leaders, etc.;
- interviews with leaders among displaced groups.

Survey questionnaires in sampled dwellings should include the number, age and sex of family members and the number of pregnant and lactating women. The average number of persons per dwelling visited and the total number of dwellings in the camp or settlement should be calculated.

1.5.3 Mortality

During a rapid initial assessment, and before any surveillance system can be put in place, any mortality data will of necessity be retrospective. The choice of the retrospective time period used to calculate mortality rates will depend on which critical event(s) influencing mortality have to be included in the survey estimate. It will also depend on cultural events that stand out in the memories of those interviewed. A balance must be struck between expectations of greater precision (requiring longer recall periods) and avoidance of recall bias.

The survey questionnaire should in any case capture, in a culturally sensitive way, the following:

- total deaths for given period (e.g. one week),
- deaths among those under 5 years of age for the same period,
- major causes of death.

Approximate daily death rates should be calculated daily or weekly, depending on the severity of the emergency. In the acute phase of an emergency, daily deaths rates should be calculated as follows:

- crude mortality rate: number of deaths per 10 000 people daily or weekly,
- age-specific mortality rates: number of deaths per 10 000 people in the under-5 and 5-and-over age groups daily or weekly,
- cause-specific mortality rates: number of deaths from a given cause per 10 000 people daily or weekly.

Table 1.3 **Thresholds and calculations**

Thresholds	Calculations
Crude mortality rate > 1/10 000/day: severe situation > 2/10 000/day: critical situation	$$\frac{D}{\dfrac{(N+D) + N}{2}} \times \frac{10000}{sp}$$
Under 5 mortality rate: double > 2/10 000/day: severe situation > 4/10 000/day: critical situation	average population $= \dfrac{(N+D) + N}{2}$ $D =$ number of deaths during the study period
Normal and stable situation: Developing countries: 0.6/10 000/day Industrialised countries: 0.3/10 000/day	$N =$ number of people of the sample living at the end of the study period $sp =$ study period expressed in days

The following methods can be used to collect mortality data.

- Count the number of graves: designate a single burial site for the camp or settlement monitored by grave-watchers 24 hours a day, and develop a verbal autopsy procedure for expected causes of death using standard forms.
- Check hospital/health facility records and records of organizations responsible for burial.
- Interview community leaders.

- For the collection of prospective mortality data, other methods can be used, such as mandatory registration of deaths, issuing of shrouds to families of the deceased to help ensure compliance, or employing volunteer community informants to report deaths for a defined section of the population (e.g. 50 families).

1.5.4 Morbidity

The number of cases of disease should include:

- diseases that cause substantial morbidity (i.e. diarrhoea, respiratory infections and malaria where prevalent);
- diseases that have the potential to cause epidemics (i.e. measles, cholera, meningitis and haemorrhagic fevers).

Classical sources of morbidity data are:

- patient registers and records in camp or settlement clinics, hospitals or feeding centres;
- interviews with health workers, midwives within the displaced population;
- records of local hospitals or clinics.

After the acute phase is over, a properly designed emergency surveillance system should provide more accurate morbidity data (see Chapter 3).

1.5.5 Health services and infrastructure

Access

- Access by the affected population to local, pre-existing health services.
- Ability of local health services to absorb the influx of people affected by the emergency.

Facilities

- Numbers, names and types of health facilities available, i.c. clinics, hospitals, feeding centres and laboratories.
- Level of support – ministry of health or nongovernmental organization.
- Level of functioning.
- Level of damage.
- Number of beds including maternity beds – total and occupied currently.
- Average number of outpatients seen per day – 6 months ago and current.
- Average number of deliveries during one week – 6 months ago and current.
- Availability of operating theatres.
- Numbers, type, size and capacity of health facilities set up for the displaced population if separate (e.g. tent, local materials).
- Adequacy of water supply, vaccine cold chain (freezers and refrigerators), generators or town electricity, toilets and waste disposal facilities and food for patients or malnourished.

Health personnel

- Per health facility above, types and numbers of health personnel and relevant skills and experience present in the hosting area – 6 months ago and current.
- Health workers present among the displaced population, including traditional healers, traditional midwives, doctors and nurses, laboratory technicians, and water and sanitation engineers.
- Availability of interpreters.

Drug and vaccine supplies

- Availability of essential drugs and medical supplies (see Annex 2 – Rapid Health Assessment, Table 1).
- Availability of the WHO New Emergency Health Kit, which contains drugs and medical supplies for 10 000 people for approximately 3 months (see Annex 10).
- Availability of essential vaccines and vaccination equipment (e.g. measles vaccines, injection material and cold chain equipment).

1.5.6   Food

- Number of calories available per person per day.
- Frequency of distribution of food rations.
- Length of time these rations have been provided.
- Food basket monitoring.

Sources of data

- Assessment of the quality and type of food available to the population.
- Inspection of local markets for food availability and prices.
- Assessment of local, regional and national markets for availability of appropriate emergency foods.

1.5.7   Nutritional status

(See also Section 2.5.)

- Prevalence of acute malnutrition in children 6–59 months of age or 60–110 cm in height.
- Percentage of children severely and moderately malnourished.
- Prevalence of clinically observable micronutrient deficiencies.
- Feeding programmes currently being planned – number of children being cared for daily in supplementary feeding programmes (SFP) and therapeutic feeding programmes (TFP).
- Number of additional calories per day provided by SFP.

Sources of data

- Unbiased representative sampling.
- Mass screening (all children weighed and measured).

1.5.8   Water

- Litres of water per person per day.
- Length of time this quantity has been available.
- Source and quality of water.
- Number and type of water points.
- Water storage facilities.
- Water purification methods available/in use.
- Length of time persons must wait for water.
- Number of persons per water point.
- Transport and storage.
- Equipment/expertise on site, planned or available if needed.

1.5.9   Sanitation

- Current facilities for excreta disposal and population per latrine or toilet.
- Anal cleansing methods and availability.
- Availability of soap.
- Presence of vectors (arthropods, mammals).
- Adequacy of burial sites.

1.5.10   Shelter and non-food items

- Blankets, clothing and domestic utensils.
- Shelter.
- Livestock.

1.5.11   Environment

- Climate.
- Topography and drainage.
- Suitability as site for settlement from health point of view.
- Access (routes to site, road surface, airfields, security issues).
- Transport.
- Amount of land: persons per square metre.
- Building materials.
- Fuel availability.
- Storage facilities for food, medical supplies.
- Communication.

Sources of data

- This assessment is largely carried out by visual inspection. Information must also be obtained from key informants such as local officials and United Nations, international and nongovernmental organizations.

– Focus group discussions with the community may also be useful, addressing such issues as their cultural perceptions of water and sanitation, how they bury the dead, and where they find food, fuel and shelter materials.

1.5.12 Coordination

The following information should be obtained from national, United Nations, international and nongovernmental organizations working on the affected area.

- What is the existing local response capacity?
- What is the presence and activities of international or local organizations?
- Who is in charge of coordinating health, water and sanitation activities?
- Who supplies which services in these sectors?
- Who coordinates food delivery to the area and its distribution to the affected populations?
- What have they achieved to date?
- What are the additional needs in terms of financial and material resources, and of implementation capacity?
- What are the priorities for immediate action?

A summary of the essential information to be collected during a rapid assessment is given in Table 1.4.

1.5.13 Common sources of error

Logistic
- Insufficient transport and/or fuel.
- Visas/security clearance not received in time.
- Inadequate communication between field, regional and national levels: authorities in charge not informed in time and not ready to assist.

Organizational
- Lead organization not identified, team leader not identified, responsibilities of various organizations not well defined.
- Key decision-makers and donors not informed that an assessment is being undertaken.
- Assessment conducted too late or takes too long.
- Information collected that is not needed for the emergency response.

Technical
- Specialists with appropriate skills not involved in the assessment.
- Programmes that could be implemented immediately unnecessarily delayed because of the assessment (e.g. measles vaccination).
- Assessment conclusions not representative of the affected population.
- Surveillance system developed too slowly, thus preventing monitoring and evaluation of emergency response programme.

Table 1.4	**Essential information to be collected during a rapid assessment**

- Background to the emergency
- Estimate of size of affected population and population movements
- Map of the site
- Environmental conditions
- Security conditions
- Health and nutritional status of the population affected by the emergency
- Major health threats – communicable and noncommunicable diseases
- Diseases of epidemic potential
- Existing health facilities and staff – capacity to deal with the affected population
- Estimation of recent mortality rates
- Surveillance system in place prior to the emergency
- Availability of food and water
- Extent of involvement of the local authorities, especially the Ministry of Health
- Presence and activities of international or local organizations

1.6   Analysis and presentation of results

The rapid assessment report must be:

Clear	Decision-makers or staff of local, national and international organizations whose actions depend on the results of the rapid assessment may not be trained in epidemiology. User-friendly language and graphs make complex data and trends easier to understand.
Standardized	Results should be presented according to a standard format so they can be compared with other assessments.
Action-oriented and prioritized	Clear recommendations should be made to implementing organizations, giving highest priority needs.
Widely distributed	Copies of the report should be distributed to all organizations involved in the emergency response.
Timely	The assessment and report should be finalized and distributed as quickly as possible, preferably within 3–4 days. Donors are often under political pressure in the first few days after an emergency to demonstrate support by their government and have access to funds. They must have data to base their decisions on funding priorities.

1.6.1 Further reading

Assefa F et al. Malnutrition and mortality in Kohistan district, Afghanistan, April 2001. *Journal of the American Medical Association,* 2001, **286:**2723–2728.

Gessner BD. Mortality rates, causes of death, and health status among displaced and resident populations of Kabul, Afghanistan. *Journal of the American Medical Association,* 1994, **272:**382–385.

Epi Info. Centers for Diseases Control and Prevention, Atlanta, GA, USA. Available from *http//www.cdc.gov/epiinfo*.

EpiData. The EpiData Association, Odense, Denmark. Available from *http://www. epidata.dk*.

Henderson RH, Sundaresan T. Cluster sampling to assess vaccination coverage: a review of experience with a simplified sampling method. *Bulletin of the World Health Organization*, 1982, **60:**253–260.

Lwanga SK, Lemeshow S. *Sample size determination in health studies: a practical manual*. Geneva, World Health Organization, 1991.

Malilay J, Flanders WD, Brogan D. A modified cluster-sampling method for post-disaster rapid assessment of needs. *Bulletin of the World Health Organization*, 1996, **74:**399–405.

Porter JDH, van Look FL, Devaux A. Evaluation of two Kurdish refugee camps in Iran, May 1991: the value of cluster sampling in producing priorities and policy. *Disasters*, 1993, **17:**341–347.

Rapid health assessment protocols for emergencies. Geneva, World Health Organization, 1999.

Roberts L, Despines M. Mortality in eastern Democratic Republic of Congo. *Lancet*, 1999, **353**(9171):2249–2250.

Roberts L. *Mortality in eastern Democratic Republic of Congo: results from eleven mortality surveys*. Final draft. New York, International Rescue Committee, 2001. *http://intranet.theirc.org/docs/mortII_report_small.pdf*
http://intranet.theirc.org/docs/mortII_graphs.pdf
http://intranet.theirc.org/docs/mortII_map.pdf
http://intranet.theirc.org/docs/mortII_exec.pdf

Rothenberg RB et al. Observations on the application EPI cluster survey methods for estimating disease incidence. *Bulletin of the World Health Organization*, 1985, **63:**93–99

2. PREVENTION

This includes good site planning; provision of basic clinical services, shelter, clean water and proper sanitation; mass vaccination against specific diseases; a regular and sufficient food supply; and control of disease vectors. Table 2.1 lists the main diseases and disease groups targeted by such interventions.

Table 2.1 **Diseases targeted by preventive measures**

Preventive measure	Impact on spread of:
Site planning	diarrhoeal diseases, acute respiratory infections
Clean water	diarrhoeal diseases, typhoid fever, guinea worm
Good sanitation	diarrhoeal diseases, vector-borne diseases, scabies
Adequate nutrition	tuberculosis, measles, acute respiratory infections
Vaccination	measles, meningitis, yellow fever, Japanese encephalitis, diphtheria
Vector control	malaria, plague, dengue, Japanese encephalitis, yellow fever, other viral haemorrhagic fevers
Personal protection (insecticide-treated nets)	malaria, leishmaniasis
Personal hygiene	louse-borne diseases: typhus, relapsing fever, trench fever
Health education	sexually transmitted infections, HIV/AIDS, diarrhoeal diseases
Case management	cholera, shigellosis, tuberculosis, acute respiratory infections, malaria, dengue haemorrhagic fever, meningitis, typhus, relapsing fever

2.1 Shelter

In many emergency situations, the displaced population must be sheltered in temporary settlements or camps. The selection of sites must be well planned to avoid risk factors for communicable disease transmission, such as overcrowding, poor hygiene, vector breeding sites and lack of adequate shelter. Such conditions favour the transmission of diseases such as measles, meningitis and cholera. Usually, the most suitable land is already occupied by the local population, leaving less desirable areas available to refugees or displaced people. Critical factors to consider when planning a site are: water availability, means of transport, access to fuel, access to fertile soil and for security reasons, a sufficient distance from national borders or frontlines.

The surrounding environment may also pose a threat to health in the form of vectors not encountered in the population's previous place of residence. In order to reduce such risks it is essential that site selection, planning and organization be undertaken as soon as possible.

2.1.1   Site selection criteria

Settlements should avoid the major breeding sites of local vectors, as well as marshy areas and flat, low-lying ground at risk of flooding. Preference should be given to gently sloping, well drained sites on fertile soil with tree cover, sheltered from strong winds. Local expertise and knowledge of the biology of the vectors should be considered, such as avoiding forested hills in some Asian countries where vectors proliferate. If not already sufficiently documented by national and local health services, the epidemiological characteristics of the area need to be assessed quickly.

The following criteria should be considered when assessing site suitability; other criteria may also be relevant in specific situations.

Water supply

The availability of an adequate amount of safe water throughout the year has proved in practice to be the single most important criterion for site location. The water source should be close enough to avoid transporting water by trucks, pumping it over long distances or walking long distances to collect insufficient quantities.

Space

There must be enough space for the present number of emergency-affected population, with provision for future influxes and for amenities such as water and sanitation facilities, food distribution centres, storage sites, hospitals, clinics and reception centres.

Topography and drainage

Gently sloping sites above the flood level is preferred in order to provide natural drainage. Flat areas, depressions, swamp, river banks and lakeshore sites should be avoided. Windy sites are unsuitable, as temporary shelters are usually fragile.

Soil conditions

The soil type affects sanitation, water pipelines, road and building construction, drainage and the living environment (in terms of dust and mud). The most suitable soil type is one that will easily absorb human waste.

Access

The site should be accessible at all times (e.g. for food deliveries, roads during rains).

Vegetation

The site area should have good vegetation cover if possible. Trees and plants provide shade, help to prevent soil erosion, allow recharge of the groundwater supplies and help in reducing dust. It may sometimes be necessary, however, to destroy poisonous trees or plants, for example where populations are accustomed to collecting berries or mushrooms.

Environmental health

Areas near vector breeding sites where there is a risk of contracting malaria, onchocerciasis (river blindness), schistosomiasis, trypanosomiasis, etc. should be avoided.

Security

The site chosen should be in a safe area, sufficiently distant from national borders and combat areas.

Local population

The use of land for a camp can cause friction with local farmers, herdsmen, nomads and landowners. Some potential sites may have special ritual or spiritual significance to local people, and site selection must respect the wishes of the local population. Streams or rivers used for bathing and laundry may cause pollution far downstream; water abstraction will reduce flow rates. Indiscriminate defecation in the early stages may also pollute water supplies used by the local population.

Fuel supply

Fuel for cooking is an essential daily requirement. Options for fuel include wood, charcoal and kerosene. In practice, wood from surrounding forests is the most likely fuel. It is important to liaise closely with the local forestry department to control indiscriminate felling and collection.

2.1.2   Site layout and design

It is important to prepare a master plan of the camp. The site plan should be sufficiently flexible to allow for a greater than expected influx of people. A 3–4% per year population growth rate must also be planned for.

Overdevelopment of some areas of the site must be avoided as it can cause health problems, especially for people who come from sparsely populated environments.

Tribal, ethnic or religious differences may exist within the camp population or between this population and the local people, or such groupings may develop or be strengthened with time. The camp must be planned in such a way that these divisions are honoured.

Site planning norms are presented in Table 2.2. The recommended figures for camp layout and services are only guidelines. In severely overcrowded, spontaneously settled camps it may be very difficult to achieve the recommended figures during the initial emergency phase and realistic compromises will have to be made. Nevertheless, the figures provide the basis for planning and are the targets at which to aim.

Table 2.2   **Site planning norms**

Area per person for collective activities	30 m^2 [a]
Shelter space per person	3.5 m^2 [b] (4.5–5.5 m^2 [c] in cold climates)
Distance between shelters	2 m minimum
Area for support services	7.5 m^2/person
Number of people per water point	250
Number of people per latrine	20
Distance to water point	150 m maximum
Distance to latrine	30 m
Distance between water point and latrine	100 m
Firebreaks	75 m every 300 m

[a] *In practice this may be difficult to achieve, for example in areas with a high population density where little land is available. This figure includes roads, services, shelter, etc. but depends on the layout and terrain. It does not include land for livestock or agriculture. After space for covered shelter and support services, the remainder of the 30 m^2/person area is for family plot space, latrines, washing and cooking areas, community space, roads, firebreaks, drainage, burial grounds and contingencies.*

[b] *For a five-person family this equals a shelter 6 by 3 metres in a plot 15 by 10 metres.*

[c] *In cold climates where cooking is done indoors, extra shelter space is required.*

2.1.3   Community participation

Ongoing community involvement in site planning and management is crucial and can maximize the effectiveness of the intervention.

2.1.4   Location of family dwellings

The layout of dwellings relative to each other can have a significant impact on security and cultural activities, and is important for the building of a social structure. It also affects the use of latrines and water points. Although shelters arranged in straight lines on a close grid pattern might appear to ease some aspects of camp management, such a pattern is not normally conducive to social cohesion. The camp should be organized into small community units or "villages" each of approximately 1000 people. Traditional living patterns should always be taken into account. Several villages can be combined to form a group; several groups can form a section; and there can be several sections in one camp. Table 2.3 shows the recommended structural organization for a camp setting. Each group or section will require a number of decentralized services, which are listed in Table 2.4.

The grouping of family plots into community units provides a defined, secure space within each unit. People know each other and strangers will stand out. The circumstances of an emergency may give rise to additional personal security risks. Women may be vulnerable to harassment and rape. Ethnic and factional divisions can provoke violent confrontations. In these circumstances the protection aspects of "shelter"' may mean keeping different refugee groups apart and/or the provision of secure compounds for particularly vulnerable refugees.

Table 2.3 **Camp building blocks**

1 family	= 4–6 people	
16 families	= 80 people	= 1 community
16 communities	= 1250 people	= 1 block
4 blocks	= 5000 people	= 1 sector
4 sectors	= 20 000 people	= 1 camp

2.1.5   Shelter design

A minimum shelter space of 3.5 m² per person is recommended in emergency situations. If possible, the emergency-affected population should build their own shelters, preferably using local materials such as timber, grass, bamboo, mud, sand and woven mats. Woven matting, natural fibre screens and bamboo make very good ventilated walls. When necessary, rolled-up plastic sheeting can be let down to make these walls water-, draught- and dust-proof. Tents and plastic sheeting provide reasonable protection from the elements, but with large numbers of people many units are required. Plastic sheeting may last only 6–9 months, depending on the quality used; it degrades as a result of exposure to the elements, especially sunlight. Canvas tents can last for up to two years if well maintained. The build-up of dirt or rainwater on the roof, or dirt on the walls, will shorten the life of a canvas tent.

It is best to plan the layout of shelter areas in community clusters adjacent to the relevant latrines, water points and washing areas. These community units should be as close as possible in design and layout to those with which the population is most familiar.

2.1.6   Location of site services

Consideration must be given to the location of roads, houses, food and water distribution points, emergency services (security, fire, medical), drains, washing areas, latrines and solid waste pits. Public buildings require access roads for vehicles and should be centrally located where possible.

Food distribution centres must be centrally located, with sufficient room for crowds of people waiting and for trucks delivering food. Good design can help considerably in crowd control and theft prevention. The main health facility must be in a safe and accessible place, preferably on the periphery of the site to allow for future expansion and to avoid overcrowding.

A site for a cholera treatment centre must be identified in advance, separate from other health facilities and in an area where water supplies cannot be contaminated.

Support facilities must be located away from dusty or potentially dangerous major access roads.

Table 2.4   **Main facilities on settlements**

Centralized	Decentralized
Administration	Community health centres
Coordination offices	Bathing and washing areas
Warehouse	Social centres
Registration	Schools
Hospital (for large camps)	Recreation space
Tracing centres	Supplementary feeding centres
Therapeutic feeding centres	Religious buildings
Food distribution centres	Water points
Training centres	Latrines
	Sanitation offices
	Roads and firebreaks
	Markets

2.1.7   Reception and registration

A reception area must be set up outside the settlement to receive and register new arrivals before they become integrated within the camp. The registration site should preferably be a large, flat, open space with a water supply and latrines or defecation areas. Temporary first-night shelter and land for accompanying animals may be needed.

2.1.8   Markets

Market areas are important trading and social centres, but they can pose health risks where food and drink is for sale. The planning and layout of such areas are very important. If possible the market should be outside the camp, or several small market areas can be established. Vector control, waste collection and disposal measures need to be particularly stringent at market areas.

Markets must be divided into food and non-food areas. Food areas should be further divided into areas for raw and processed foods.

Areas must be provided for the slaughter of livestock, if possible with a concrete slab with good drainage to carry away blood and animal droppings (although one needs to ensure that this does not drain directly into a watercourse).

2.1.9   Noise avoidance and traffic

Generators and pumps should be located away from family dwellings and the buildings housing them should be soundproofed, with sufficient ventilation for the escape of exhaust fumes. Traffic should be limited to main routes.

2.1.10   Camp coordination

Coordination between the various organizations working in the emergency is essential in order to maximize positive impact on the population by means of effective management and integration of relief activities.

The following steps are necessary to achieve this objective:

- establish clear leadership,
- create a coordinating body,
- ensure that programme activities are shared by agencies,
- clarify the roles and responsibilities of all partners,
- prevent duplication of activities,
- establish good communication channels,
- ensure that all needs are addressed,
- create and implement agreed common policies, standards and guidelines.

2.1.11   Liaison with local communities

Continued liaison with local communities is essential. The influx of emergency-affected populations into their area means that they are now affected by the emergency. There is a real risk of generating resentment if local people feel that the emergency-affected populations are better served than they are. There may be a need to provide medical or other assistance to local communities, both to ensure equity and to prevent the spread of disease.

2.2   Water

Water and sanitation are vital elements in the transmission of communicable diseases and in the spread of diseases prone to cause epidemics. Diarrhoeal diseases are a major cause of morbidity and mortality among emergency-affected populations, most being caused by a lack of safe water, inadequate excreta disposal facilities and poor hygiene (see Table 2.5).

The goal of a water and sanitation programme is to minimize risks to the health of a population, particularly one caught up in the difficult circumstances of an emergency with its attendant displacement and dangers. Such a programme is an integral part of preventive health activities.

The main focus of such a programme is on:

- the provision of a safe and sufficient water supply,

- provision for excreta disposal and the establishment of other waste control and hygiene measures,
- a programme of public education for the affected population on the issues of hygiene and water use.

Table 2.5 **Water-related diseases**

Diseases that occur owing to a lack of water and poor personal hygiene	Skin infections: scabies, impetigo
	Ophthalmic infections: conjunctivitis, trachoma
	Louse-borne diseases: typhus, relapsing fever, trench fever
Diseases that occur owing to poor biological quality of the water	Caused by faecal pollution: cholera, typhoid, other diarrhoeal diseases, hepatitis A, hepatitis E, schistosomiasis
	Caused by the urine of certain mammals: leptospirosis
Conditions that occur owing to poor chemical quality of the water	Poisoning
Diseases caused by water-based insect vectors	Malaria, dengue fever, onchocerciasis, yellow fever, Japanese encephalitis, guinea worm

In an emergency, the affected populations need immediate access to a water supply in order to maintain health and to reduce the risk of epidemics. If the emergency-affected population have to be sheltered in temporary settlements or camps, water supply is an essential consideration in choosing the site location. An adequate amount of safe drinking-water must be provided for the entire displaced population.

The first objective is to provide sufficient water; quality can be addressed later. Sufficient water of low quality is better than very little water of high quality. During the rapid assessment of a proposed site it is essential to protect existing water sources from possible contamination. If the population have already moved into the area in question, then immediate measures should be taken to isolate and protect the water source, if it is on or near the site.

Essential water requirements

- The minimum amount of water required in extreme situations is 7 litres per person per day (only tolerable for a short duration). This amount does not reduce the risk of epidemics in the population as it permits only a very low level of hygiene.
- The emergency requirement guideline is 20 litres per person per day. This allows for cooking, laundry, bathing and activities essential to preventing the transmission of water-borne diseases.

2.2.1   Guidelines for assessing the volume of water required

The assessment of the volume of water required must take into account daily population requirements and the effects of climate on the water source. The effects on water requirements of a change in population size also need to be estimated. A factor of 10–15% should be added to the total daily requirement of a camp in order to provide for public institutions. Table 2.6 details the water requirements in health facilities.

Table 2.6   **Water requirements in health facilities**

Hospital ward	50 litres/person per day
Surgery/maternity	100 litres/person per day
Dressing/consultation	5 litres per dressing
Feeding centre	20–30 litres/person per day
Kitchen	10 litres/person per day

When water is scarce, rationing should be introduced to ensure that the weak and vulnerable survive and that an equitable distribution is achieved. In this situation, monitoring is essential.

2.2.2   Providing a water supply

Identification of possible sources

The affected population must be involved in this process from the start, as they will be relied on for repairs and maintenance in the future. All available sources of water should be considered: a combination of sources may be used.

Assessment of water sources

Assessment is needed to determine:

* the quality of the water,
* the type of treatment needed,
* the method of extraction from the source,
* the most suitable distribution system.

Water quality

The key to disease prevention through water supply is ensuring that water is of a high quality when consumed, not only just after treatment or at distribution points. If people do not have enough water of acceptable quality, then they will take water from other sources, which will most likely be contaminated.

In an emergency, biological quality is of greater importance than chemical quality. The WHO guidelines detailed in Table 2.7 list the basic requirements and parameters that must be measured. Groundwater sources usually yield water of good quality, but chemicals that produce a bad odour or taste may also be released into the water from underlying rocks.

Table 2.7   **WHO guidelines on water quality**

Criteria	Guidelines
Faecal coliforms [a]	< 10 per 100 ml
Odour/taste	not detectable
Turbidity [b]	< 5 NTU
Total dissolved solids [c]	< 500 parts per million
pH [d]	6.5–8.5

[a] *Faecal coliforms are bacteria of faecal origin from the faeces of an animal (including humans). This parameter is the most important when testing water for drinking. Fewer than 10 coliforms per 100 ml of water is acceptable. The preferred level is zero, but this may not be practical in some cases.*

[b] *Turbidity refers to water clarity. It is measured in "nephelometric turbidity units" (NTU). Turbidity may only be of aesthetic importance, but this will matter to the affected population. It does inhibit the effectiveness of chlorine in purifying the water and may also be an indication of the level of pollution.*

[c] *Total dissolved solids refers to the quantity of dissolved matter in the water. It is measured in parts per million (ppm). Drinking-water should have less than 500 ppm. Again, this relates to acceptability by the consumers.*

[d] *pH is a measure of the acidity or alkalinity of the water. Alum (aluminium sulfate, used in the flocculation of suspended solids) works more efficiently at a pH between 6 and 8. The pH should be less than 7 before adding chlorine. Lime can be added to raise the pH and hydrochloric acid to lower it.*

Water treatment

Water that does not meet the required standards must be treated before it is distributed to the population. Table 2.8 presents the main methods of water treatment, the selection of which depends on the extent and type of purification required. Treatment is usually followed by chemical disinfection of the water, the most common and effective disinfecting solution in emergency situations being chlorine (see Table 2.9).

Quality control

Water quality checks must be made at regular intervals throughout all stages of the water distribution chain. Tests are needed several times a day at the beginning and in the middle of the chain for free residual chlorine. Weekly checks for faecal coliforms are needed in emergency situations, and particularly during epidemics.

Distribution

If the rapid assessment indicates that a suitable water system will take some time to develop, short-term measures such as trucking may have to be considered. In such instances, rationing may be necessary to ensure equal distribution among the entire population.

Once a satisfactory supply has been established, enough storage and reserve systems must be developed to allow for maintenance and breakdowns in supply and equipment. Storage of at least one day's requirement must be provided. Preventing contamination from sanitation facilities and other sources of pollution is of paramount importance. The location, organization and maintenance of water points is detailed in Table 2.10.

Table 2.8	Methods of water treatment
Storage	This is the simplest method of improving water quality. If water is stored in a covered tank for a period of time, pathogenic bacteria die off and sink to the bottom by a simple sedimentation process. Two days is the minimum length of storage recommended. The water will not necessarily be totally free of contamination by simple filtration.
	Storage tanks require cleaning and de-sludging at regular intervals, depending on the level of sediment in the water. Algal build-up should be prevented. No animals or unauthorized persons should be allowed access to the tanks.
Aeration	Aeration is achieved by allowing the water to cascade over layers of gravel. Aeration may be required if iron or manganese is present in the water, since these give an unpleasant taste and a brownish discoloration to food and clothes.
Sedimentation	Water from river sources, especially in the rainy season, often has a high silt content. Simple storage methods are not sufficient for this silt to settle. Along with the natural sedimentation process, the addition of a chemical coagulant, usually aluminium sulfate (alum), is necessary.
	The amount of alum needed depends on the amount of suspended matter in the water, the turbidity, the pH and the hardness of the water. Effluent water should not contain a concentration of alum greater than the guideline figure given in the WHO guidelines for drinking-water quality.
Filtration	Slow and rapid sand filters.
Disinfection	Chlorine is the most common and effective disinfecting solution in emergency situations, and various dilutions are used in different situations (see Table 10). The amount of chlorine required depends on the quantity of organic matter and of harmful organisms in the water.
	The dose should leave a residual level of chlorine of between 0.2 and 0.5 mg/litre (a higher level will leave a taste and people will not drink the water). A simple drip-feed tank can be designed to administer the correct amount of chlorine.

Table 2.9   **Recommended dilution and use of Aquatabs®**

Tablet size	Chlorine per tablet (mg)	Clear piped water	Protected tube wells, ring wells, clear rainwater	Unprotected wells and cloudy water: filter before purifying	Water known to have faecal contamination: filter before purifying
		Volume of water treated per tablet (litres)			
8.5 mg	5	5	2.5	1	0.5
17 mg	10	10	5	2	1
67 mg	39.41	39.41	19.7	7.88	3.94
340 mg	200	200	100	40	20
500 mg	294	294	147	58.8	29.4
Free available chlorine content after treatment (residual)		1 mg/litre	2 mg/litre	5 mg/litre	10 mg/litre

Column header spanning: "Type of water and source"

Table 2.10   **Water distribution points**

Location	Water distribution points must be set up in suitable places around the camp. A good location is an elevated spot in the centre of a living area.

If the water points are from ground sources, no sanitation facilities should be within 50 metres, and definitely not closer than 30 metres. If the water point is too far away, people will not collect enough water or may use contaminated sources nearby. |
| **Design** | When designing water points consider the following:
• traditional water-carrying methods,
• the containers used: for example, a raised area is suitable for people who carry the bucket on their heads,
• who collects and carries the water (it is usually the women and children),
• the availability of spare parts.

There should be enough space on the concrete slab around the water point for laundry and bathing areas. If sanitation is compromised, it may be felt necessary to locate bathing and washing areas away from collection points. However, traditional practices and habits need to be accommodated as much as possible.

Animals must certainly be kept away. If they are mobile herds, watering facilities should be established some distance away and a fence erected around the water point. |
| **Number** | One tap per 200–250 people is the ratio recommended by the United Nations High Commissioner for Refugees (UNHCR). The more people there are per tap, the more wear and tear there is.

Nobody should have to wait longer than a few minutes; if collection takes a long time, people will return to old, contaminated but quicker sources. |

Protection	All efforts must be made to reduce contamination at the water point.
	In the case of wells, clean buckets must be provided. Ideally, the well will be sealed and a lifting device installed. There should be a concrete apron for the water point, angled so that sullage and spilt water is carried away and disposed of or used (e.g. in a soakaway pit or vegetable garden). Standing water around a water point will become contaminated, attract animals, make the apron muddy and provide a breeding site for mosquitoes. It can also seep back into the water source and contaminate it.
Maintenance	Each water point must have a caretaker to look after it, keep it clean and make sure it is not abused (women are usually the most appropriate caretakers; in the long term they must be trained in maintenance skills). Caretakers must live close to the water point.

Domestic storage

It is important to provide clean storage containers for use in the home. Providing high-quality water at a tap-stand is of little impact if people are unable to carry and store that water hygienically or do not appreciate the importance of this. Intensive education will improve hygiene practices.

In the acute phase of an emergency, household storage is likely to be in plastic containers. People may use a plastic jerrycan for carrying and storing water and a bucket for washing. Closed jerrycans of 10–20 litres capacity are ideal as they can be carried by children. Vegetable oil is often distributed in this type of container, and they can be used for water when empty. If possible, large containers (100–200 litres) with lids should be made available. These allow for the safe storage of water, plus a reserve to cope with a short break in supply.

Water can also be stored in concrete storage jars that can be made on site. These jars improve storage and, in addition, the skills learned in making the jars can be used when the emergency is over. It is essential that any water container is kept clean and covered.

2.2.3 Further reading

Davis J, Lambert R. *Engineering in emergencies: a practical guide for relief workers*, 2nd ed. London, ITDG Publishing, 2002.

House SJ, Reed RA. *Emergency water sources: guidelines for selection and treatment*. Loughborough, Water, Engineering and Development Centre, 1997.

Public health engineering in emergency situations. Paris, Médecins Sans Frontières, 1994.

Smout, IK, ed. *Guidance manual on water supply and sanitation programmes*. Loughborough, Water, Engineering and Development Centre, 1998.

Water manual for refugee situations. Geneva, Office of the United Nations High Commissioner for Refugees, 1992.

2.3   Sanitation

The aim of a sanitation programme is to develop physical barriers against the transmission of disease, in order to protect the health of the emergency-affected population. These barriers include both engineering measures and personal hygiene measures. The provision of latrines and the development of methods of waste disposal are essential elements of the programme. These measures are only fully effective, however, when complemented by a sanitation education programme.

2.3.1   Waste disposal: human waste

The efficient and safe disposal of human excreta is as important as the provision of water in its positive effect on the health of the emergency-affected population. Human excreta is more likely to transmit disease than animal waste. It contributes to the transmission of numerous diseases (which can be particularly when combined with low levels of nutrition) and can also be a breeding ground for flies and other insects. In the acute phase of an emergency, any form of excreta disposal is better than none. The simplest and quickest methods should be adopted; these can later be improved on and changed. Initially, speedy action is important in averting human catastrophe.

Immediate action

Excretion fields must be prepared on the first day.

Indiscriminate defaecation needs to be controlled. Areas where defaecation cannot be permitted are:

* near rivers, streams and lakes and within 30 metres of any water source or water point,
* near water storage facilities,
* uphill of the camp,
* uphill of water sources,
* along public roads,
* near feeding centres, clinics, food storage depots and distribution centres.

These areas should be fenced off and guarded where necessary. The use of water for anal cleansing may explain defaecation near water sources. Water must be provided in alternative locations to control this practice effectively. These measures must be announced throughout the camp with the assistance of the community leaders, and displayed on signs, using both words and pictures.

Latrine design

The most common cause of failure of a sanitation system is the selection of the wrong system of latrines for a given situation. As potential latrine users will be relied on for inspection and maintenance, it is essential that they be involved from the beginning in planning, design and implementation. This should ensure the most appropriate latrine design for the custom and culture of the population.

In designing the system, the requirements of women, young children and people with disabilities need to be considered.

Education and promotion

Where it is necessary to introduce unfamiliar types of latrines, the emergency-affected population may need training in the proper use of the system.

Where acceptable latrines are provided, intensive education and promotion is still needed to maximize the numbers of displaced persons using them. This is especially important for the children, who may not have used latrines before.

The design of latrines should be such as to encourage children to use them. Babies will not use latrines, and their faeces are more dangerous than those of an adult. Mothers should be encouraged to dig small holes for their babies' faeces and to cover them with soil afterwards.

The digging of latrine pits must begin as soon as possible. A complete camp coverage of one latrine per 50 people should be the first target; then one per four families; and finally one per family. Funding or space constraints may hinder reaching the highest ratios. Often the best ratio achieved in an emergency situation is one latrine per four families.

Appropriate anal cleansing facilities must be provided.

2.3.2   Waste disposal: solid waste

Solid waste, if not properly disposed of, acts as a breeding site for flies, cockroaches and rats. A system for the safe storage, collection and disposal of waste must be implemented in the earliest stages of an emergency. Consultation with the emergency-affected population is very important, as they may already be motivated to carry out some of the necessary tasks without outside intervention, and may also want to use their waste in a constructive way (e.g. in compost production). Table 2.11 summarizes the options for solid waste disposal.

Every household must be no more than 15 metres away from a refuse container, with one waste container for ten houses. Old oil drums cut in half are often used as receptacles. They must be covered or set above animal foraging height. Holes drilled in the bottom allow liquids to drain away and also prevent them from being stolen and used as water storage containers. Containers must be properly secured.

Table 2.11   **Options for solid waste disposal**

Burial of family waste near the home	In a settlement with sufficient space, the population can be encouraged to dispose of their waste within their own plots. A small hole can be dug and the waste, if dry enough, can be burned before burying.
Transport of waste by householders to a community compost pit	If the affected population are interested or experienced in composting their waste, compost pits can make a very efficient disposal system. They must be well managed in order to keep the fly population down. If the pits are small enough to be located at various sites throughout the camp, there may be no need for solid waste collection.
	If the population understand the dangers of flies and rats they will be more inclined to manage the compost heap correctly. They may also be motivated by the possibility of utilizing or selling the compost.
Waste collection near homes and transfer to large disposal site	The most expensive option; often the only solution in large, overcrowded settlements.

2.3.3   Waste disposal: liquid waste

Sullage is wastewater from bathing, laundry and food preparation. It must be drained away as it attracts flies and mosquitoes and can contaminate water supplies. Sullage also provides a breeding ground for *Culex* mosquitoes, vectors of filariasis, Japanese encephalitis, and other vector-borne diseases.

People tend to do their washing and bathing close to the water source, such as a river or lake, unless alternative facilities are provided. This adds to the water pollution problems in the camp. Separate areas must be provided for laundry and bathing.

A washing area consists of a raised concrete platform and a drainage system. If water is in short supply, water distribution points can be linked to laundry areas as spillage at tap stands can be drained to the clothes-washing area. Laundry washing water needs to be drained carefully since it contains a large amount of phosphates and should not be directed toward water sources.

Wastewater from bathing can be dealt with easily. There is no need for a roof on a shower room, although a screen-like superstructure is necessary. If the sun dries the room each day then any pathogens existing in stagnant water will be killed off.

Sullage can be channelled into the storm-water drains, but this will not be washed away in the dry season. If the sullage cannot be drained away it may be necessary to divert it into a soakaway or a waste stabilization pond.

2.3.4   Waste disposal: medical waste

Medical waste includes needles, scalpels, laboratory samples, disposable materials stained with body fluids, and body tissue. This waste requires special care in handling, since needles and scalpels can cut handlers and transmit diseases such as HIV/AIDS, hepatitis B and C and viral haemorrhagic fevers.

Medical waste should be burnt in an incinerator, preferably as close as possible to the source, e.g. within the clinic or hospital grounds, but also downwind of hospital buildings and dwellings.

In temporary situations, a 200-litre drum can be used as an incinerator, divided in half by a metal grate and with an access hole at the bottom to provide air for combustion and as a way of removing ash.

In hospitals where there is no incinerator, placenta pits can be used for human tissues. Organic waste such as placentas and amputated limbs can be burned and then buried deep within these pits, although measures should be taken to ensure that the groundwater will not be contaminated.

At small medical facilities such as clinics, a small hole 1 m × 1 m × 1 m can be dug for the burning and burial of hazardous waste, such as syringes and soiled dressings.

Great care should be taken with sharp materials such as broken glass, scalpels and old syringes. They should be placed within old metal containers (cooking oil or milk powder tins) that are sealed before burial (see safe disposal of needles in Section 2.6.2).

2.3.5   Dust

Large amounts of dust can also be a health hazard, causing respiratory problems and contaminating food. Preventing the destruction of vegetation is important in controlling dust. Settlements with little or no vegetation are not only dusty but are also full of rubbish blown from disposal sites. Dust can be settled by spraying water on the ground: this is particularly useful around health centres and feeding centres.

2.3.6   Disposal of the dead

The risks posed by the dead are of two types: risks to those handling the cadaver, and risks to the population in general.

In the majority of cases dead bodies do not pose a serious health risk. The diseased living are a far greater hazard than the deceased, because most pathogens do not long survive the chemical and temperature changes that occur after the death of their host. Even if they do survive, the conditions suitable for multiplication of the organisms are rarely met. In the living, organisms multiply and are readily transmitted.

When death has been due to a highly infectious disease such as cholera, typhus, plague or viral haemorrhagic fever, it may be necessary to dispose of the body as quickly as possible.

In the case of cholera, bodies should be disinfected with a 2% chlorine solution and the orifices blocked with cotton wool soaked in chlorine solution; they must then be buried in plastic sacks as soon as possible.

Those who have died of typhus should be bagged as soon as possible to prevent the migration of lice to others. Ideally the cadavers should be treated with insecticide.

Individuals who have died of viral haemorrhagic fever should be handled with full biohazard precautions, wrapped in sealed leakproof material (body bag) immediately, and either be cremated or buried at a depth of at least 2 metres. If body bags are not available, wrapping the corpse in a fabric soaked in a disinfectant such as formaldehyde, then covering with a plastic sheet and sealing in a plastic bag, is recommended. The clothing, bedding and other belongings of the individual should be burned.

The use of chloride of lime should be avoided. It generally has little effect on the disease risk as it is rapidly neutralized and it presents a hazard to the handlers.

Ideally the method of disposal should follow the cultural practices of the population of which the deceased was a member. In the acute phase of an emergency, where many deaths have occurred, there may be pressure to conduct mass burials. However, this should be avoided if at all possible, to ensure relatives of the deceased have the opportunity to identify the bodies and allow burial in a marked site. Burial sites must be identified early on, and the site should ideally be located at the outskirts of the settlement (or community) and away from water sources.

During an outbreak with a high mortality rate, the collection of bodies and their rapid burial is a priority. Corpses should not be embalmed but buried or cremated promptly. With a large number of bodies there is not enough time to undertake the normal ceremonies of burial. Individual cremation is rarely possible owing to shortages of fuel. Everything should be done to try to record the names of the dead and the number of bodies interred. If possible, a culturally appropriate ceremony should be held at the end of the epidemic.

Graveyard and crematorium attendants should be in place to record the name, age, gender, and address of the deceased, the cause of death, the plot space used and the depth of burial. Records on the cause of death can be compiled to draw up a picture of the health problems in a camp.

Bodies should be covered by at least one meter of earth. If a mound is made over a shallow burial, there should be at least one meter between the edge of the mound and the cadaver. The reason for this is to prevent access by carrion feeders (such as jackals) or rodents (many species can burrow at least two feet) and also to prevent access by burrowing flies, some of which can dig down at least 45 cm. Where soil conditions allow digging to a sufficient depth, each burial plot can be used to contain up to three bodies, provided that: 12 months elapses between burials; there is a 30-cm gap between corpses; and the last corpse buried is a minimum of 1 metre below the surface.

2.3.7   Monitoring and evaluation of water and sanitation programmes

The major components of the water and sanitation programmes must be monitored and evaluated at regular intervals in order to assess their effectiveness and suitability. Problems identified can be addressed by means of changes in design, location or improved education methods. Monitoring is essential in ensuring that all sectors of the population receive an adequate water supply. Water shortages may result from:

- an underestimation of population size,
- the more powerful groups in the community taking more than their share,
- wastage and losses,
- a combination of these factors.

The information in Tables 2.12 and 2.13 provide baseline issues for monitoring and evaluation in water and sanitation programmes.

Table 2.12   **Indicators for monitoring interventions that provide clean water, drainage and waste disposal**

Water storage and use	Water supply	Drainage	Waste disposal
Sources of water for the population	Total population	Drainage from all water outlets	Methods of waste disposal used
Purposes for which water is used	Total number of families	Type of drainage	Intervals of waste disposal
Water collection and storage methods	Litres provided per person per day	Means of maintenance	Method of medical waste disposal (pit, incineration)
Access to stored water	Type and quality of protection of water sources	Blockages	Community involvement
Harmful practices and proposed solutions	Water distribution methods	Presence of stagnant pools of water in the camp, their location and origin	Dependence of community on external assistance for dumping
	Type and quality of protection of water outlets	Means of rainwater drainage	Cleanliness of the general area around each shelter
	Quantity of water collected per capita	Harvesting of rainwater and means	Cleanliness of market site
	Method of water disinfection		
	Number of water outlets		
	Number of functioning water outlets		
	Number of functioning water outlets protected		
	Ratio of laundry areas to number of families		
	Ratio of bathing areas to total population		
	Quantity of water wasted (amount and expressed as a percentage)		

Table 2.13   Indicators for monitoring interventions that provide sanitary latrine programmes

Latrine provision	Knowledge, attitudes and practice in relation to latrines
Number of families in the area Number of functioning latrines at the beginning of the reporting period Number of latrines built during the reporting period Number of latrines repaired during the reporting period Number of latrines reported as out of order during the reporting period Number of latrines functioning at the end of the reporting period Percentage of the population with access to functioning latrines	People using and not using latrines? Reason for use of latrines? Reasons for non-usage of latrines? Perceived benefits of the latrines Perceived problems with the latrines Users' opinions on how latrines should be used and maintained

2.3.8   Further reading

Davis J, Lambert R. *Engineering in emergencies: a practical guide for relief workers*, 2nd ed. London, ITDG Publishing, 2002.

Harvey PA, Baghri S, Reed RA. *Emergency sanitation: assessment and programme design*. Loughborough, Water, Engineering and Development Centre, 2002.

Public health engineering in emergency situations. Paris, Médecins Sans Frontières, 1994.

Smout, IK, ed. *Guidance manual on water supply and sanitation programmes*. Loughborough, Water, Engineering and Development Centre, 1998.

2.4   Vector control

The objective of this section is to provide a basic understanding of vector control in emergency situations. The purpose of a vector control programme is to reduce disease transmission by rendering the environment unfavourable for the development and survival of the vector. Prevention is better than cure, and when the planning and construction of camps is undertaken, preventing the development of vector problems should be taken into account. Complete eradication of a vector is rarely possible nor necessarily desirable, but the vector population and its life expectancy should be kept to a minimum. Community adhesion and participation in a vector control programme is essential for its success. Early diagnostic and treatment are needed to prevent severe forms of the disease (especially for malaria) when transmission control is needed to reduce incidence. Both are complementary and two essential components of any effective vector borne disease control programme.

The major biological vectors are mosquitoes, sand flies, triatomine bugs, tsetse flies, blackflies, ticks, fleas, lice, mites. Important carrier reservoirs or intermediary hosts are synanthropic flies, snails and rodents.

The diseases most commonly spread by vectors are malaria, filariasis, dengue fever, yellow fever, leishmaniasis, Chagas disease, sleeping sickness, onchocerciasis, borreliosis, typhus, and plague. Major diseases transmitted by intermediate hosts or carriers are schistosomiasis, diarrhoeal diseases and trachoma.

The main methods of vector prevention and control can be classified as personal protection; environmental control; campsite, shelter and food store sanitation; community awareness; and chemical control such as residual or space spraying, insecticide-treated traps, selective larviciding and the use of rodenticides. Vector control is very specific to the ecology of the vector, the epidemiology of the disease, the human and social environment as well as resources locally available (e.g. technical staff, structures, logistics).

It is important to seek the advice of an entomologist/environmental hygienist when designing a vector control programme. This person will assist by:

- identifying the vectors responsible for local transmission of disease,
- determining the factors that influence transmission,
- locating breeding grounds, and adult resting habits,
- deciding which control measures need to be implemented,
- deciding which specific chemical control measures to use,
- deciding which chemicals to use,
- deciding the method and interval of application,
- deciding the time and place of application,
- deciding the safety precautions necessary in the storage and use of hazardous chemicals.

2.4.1 Major arthropod vectors and associated diseases

Care should be taken to ensure that any insecticides, rodenticides, etc. that are used in control activities are registered for use in the relevant countries or that permission to use them is obtained from the appropriate government departments.

Mosquitoes

Mosquitoes are the vectors of malaria, filariasis, dengue, Japanese encephalitis and yellow fever. Table 2.14 summarizes the associated morbidity and case fatality, and main treatment and prevention measures.

Table 2.14   **Diseases spread by mosquitoes and their treatment and prevention**

Disease	Case fatality	Treatment	Prevention
Malaria *Plasmodium falciparum*	Often fatal to non-immune people	Antimalarial drugs	• Vector control: − insecticide-treated mosquito nets − long-lasting insecticidal nets − repellents − residual spraying − environmental management • Case management: − prophylactic drugs − rapid diagnosis and effective case management Monitoring the effectiveness of control methods particularly during epidemics
P. vivax	Usually considered non-fatal		
P. ovale	Usually considered non-fatal		
P. malariae	Usually considered non-fatal		
Yellow fever	Fatal in up to 50% of cases	No specific treatment available	• Isolation of infected people • Vaccination of the population • Chemical control (larviciding + space spraying) and environmental management to limit urban breeding sites of *Aedes* spp. mosquitoes
Dengue, **Dengue haemorrhagic fever**	Non-fatal Can be fatal in 10% of cases	No specific treatment available	• Isolation of infected people • Chemical control (larviciding + space spraying) and environmental management to limit urban breeding sites of *Aedes* spp. mosquitoes
Japanese encephalitis	Fatal in 0.5–60% of cases	No specific treatment available	• Isolation of infected people • Vaccination of the population • Environmental management
Filariasis	Non-fatal, may lead to elephantiasis	Diethylcarbamazine (DEC) *or* ivermectin + albendazole	• Environmental sanitation to prevent breeding of *Culex* spp. mosquitoes in polluted waters • Treated mosquito nets and residual spraying in areas where vectors are anophelines

Female mosquitoes may feed on humans and a variety of mammals, birds and reptiles, each species having a preference for a particular source of blood. Many species feed on humans, but only some of them are vectors of the diseases mentioned in Table 2.15. Their life cycle involves four stages: egg, larva, nymph and adult. All mosquitoes lay their eggs in moist areas, but each species has a specific preference for a given type of area. The control measures should be specific to the species and their ecological preferences. Table 2.15 presents information on the biological preferences of mosquito species.

Table 2.15   **Biological information on mosquito vectors**

Vector group	Vector species	Disease	Typical breeding sites	Resting site	Trans-mission	Blood source	Dispersal range
Anophelines	*Anopheles*	malaria, filariasis, arboviruses	Natural pools of unpolluted water	Indoor/ outdoor	Evening and night	Humans and animals	1 km
Culicines	*Aedes*	filariasis, yellow fever, dengue, some viral encephalitis	Water containers, small pools of stagnant water	Indoor/ outdoor	Day	Humans and animals	0.1–0.8 km
	Culex	filariasis, some viral encephalitis	Organically polluted water or natural pools of unpolluted water	Indoor/ outdoor	Day and night	Humans and animals	0.1–0.8 km
	Mansonia	filariasis	Unpolluted water with plants	Indoor/ outdoor	Day and night	Humans and animals	0.1–0.8 km

The various options for mosquito control are outlined below in Table 2.16.

Table 2.16   **Choice of control methods for different mosquitoes**

Mosquito behaviour	Control programme	Vector species	Control of transmission	Control schedule
For all mosquitoes	Local destruction of breeding sites by drainage or filling if identifiable	Most mosquito vectors; not suitable for *An. gambiae*	Totally effective	Permanent
	Larviciding with temephos		2–3 weeks partially effective	Repeated every 1–2 weeks for *Anopheles* and every 2 months for *Aedes*
	Space spraying	All mosquitoes	Effective	Weekly
			Very effective	Daily in early mornings or evenings
	Repellents	All mosquitoes	Lasts up to 6 hours with good effectiveness	Apply daily during biting hours
Indoor biting	Screening of doors and windows in house	*Anopheles, Culex, Aedes, Mansonia*	Partially effective	Put in place when house is built, repair annually

Indoor biting at night	Mosquito nets	*Anopheles, Culex, Mansonia*	Partially effective	Proper use of well-maintained bed net, change every 2–5 years
	Insecticide-treated mosquito nets		Partially or completely effective	Net must be impregnated with permethrin every 6–12 months
Indoor resting	Indoor residual spraying	*Anopheles, Culex, Mansonia and Aedes aegypti*	2–3 weeks partially or completely effective	Every 3–6 months, before the transmission season
Mosquito larvae attach to roots of aquatic vegetation	Removal of vegetation, especially water lettuce from all standing water	*Mansonia*	Partially effective	Check possible breeding sites weekly in the growing season

Lice

There are three species of louse: head, body and pubic. Head lice are not vectors of any particular disease but cause discomfort for those infested. Body lice are vectors of typhus, relapsing fever and trench fever. Pubic lice are not disease vectors. Body lice are widespread in impoverished communities in temperate climates or in mountainous areas in tropical countries. Head lice and pubic lice are present throughout the world. Louse-borne diseases, associated morbidity and mortality, treatment and prevention are presented in Table 2.17.

Louse-borne infections are common in overcrowded situations, particularly in settlements. Lice are spread via human clothing. Control methods for lice are simple and effective and are listed in Table 2.18.

Table 2.17 **Diseases spread by lice, their treatment and prevention**

Vector	Disease	Morbidity and mortality when untreated	Treatment	Prevention
Body lice	Louse-borne typhus	Fatal in 10–40% of cases	Antimicrobial	Change of clothing
	Relapsing fever	Fatal in 2–10% of cases	Change of clothing	Delousing (details in Table 2.18)
	Trench fever	Typically non-fatal	Delousing	
Head lice	No disease			See Table 2.18
Pubic lice	No disease			

Table 2.18 **Control methods for lice**

Type	Control programme	Control of transmission
Head lice	If shaving is culturally acceptable, adults and children can shave their heads; blades can be distributed to families Pharmaceutical anti-lice insecticide lotions such as malathion or permethrin can also be used and are recommended during a mass campaign People with head lice who sleep under impregnated mosquito nets commonly lose the infestation	Delouse new arrivals
Body lice	Information programme on the dangers of body lice and proposed control methods Change all clothing Boil or steam clothing for 15 minutes Treat non-washable clothing with insecticide and repeat after 1 week Impregnate clothing with permethrin during rinsing (see below) *or* For mass campaigns, administer 50 grams of insecticidal dusting powder to each individual in the population via the neck band, waistband and sleeves, paying particular attention to seams and underwear	Delouse new arrivals Care should be taken to delouse all feverish persons as well as corpses
Pubic lice	Pharmaceutical anti-lice insecticide lotions such as malathion or permethrin	Delouse new arrivals

Impregnation of clothing with insecticides

Impregnation of clothing with permethrin or etofenprox when rinsing is an effective way of controlling arthropod ectoparasites. Permethrin is safe for this purpose, but if impregnation is carried out the same safety precautions must be used as for impregnating mosquito nets. Impregnation should be done at a central point by trained staff and not by individual families. Clothing treated in this way will retain its insecticidal properties for several washes. Avoid the use of other pyrethroids, especially the cyanopyrethroids (alpha-cypermethrin, cyfluthrin, deltamethrin, lambda-cyhalothrin), as they may cause strong skin irritation.

Application of dusts for control of body lice

Application of insecticidal dusts for louse control requires the appropriate apparatus. Simple hand-pumped dusters are available and are effective but not very rapid to use. For mass treatment, powered dusters are more effective but need to be selected carefully. Dusts can easily clog spray nozzles, especially if the air is damp. Compressed air is therefore not ideal for pressurizing such equipment. Sprayers powered by carbon dioxide have been devised but are heavy and require supplies of the gas.

Mass dusting programmes require careful planning and staff must be properly trained. The public must be informed carefully about the nature of and reasons for the programme. Staff will need good protective clothing and effective dust masks that protect the whole face.

Flies

Filth flies are considered important carriers of diarrhoeal disease and eye infections. The common filth flies are the housefly (*Musca domestica*), *M. sorbens*, and the blowfly (blue or green big flies). The housefly and *M. sorbens* are the most important in the spread of disease. The housefly is thought to be important in the spread of diarrhoea, while *M. sorbens* spreads the eye infection trachoma. The role of blowflies, proliferating in emergency settings, in the spread of disease is unknown.

Table 2.19 presents some of the diseases spread by various species of the fly family, and their associated morbidity and mortality, treatment and prevention.

Table 2.19   **Main diseases in emergency situations spread by flies and their treatment and prevention**

Disease	Morbidity and mortality when untreated	Treatment	Prevention
Diarrhoeal disease (e.g. shigellosis or salmonellosis)	1–10% fatality rate	Rehydration (antimicrobial may be needed)	Good personal and kitchen hygiene, safe water and sanitary disposal of faeces Sanitation (garbage disposal, latrines...) and fly control
Trachoma	Non-fatal – eye damage, including blindness, in severe untreated infections	Cleaning the eye Antimicrobial	Good personal hygiene Adequate supplies of soap and water for washing face and hands

The control of flies is very difficult as they have many breeding and resting sites. The control measures that can be adopted include:

- sanitation: safe faecal and garbage disposal systems,
- selective application of insecticides in garbage containers, wall and fences around latrines as well as resting site of flies,
- prompt burial of corpses,
- screens for kitchens,
- safe food storage systems,
- good personal and environmental hygiene.

Mites

Mites are associated with disease, either as vectors or as burrowers into the flesh leading to secondary infections. Scabies and jiggers are examples of burrowing infestations. The trombiculid mite is the vector for scrub typhus. Its breeds in vegetation and transmission occurs during the day. Scabies is the main mite infestation seen in refugee situations. Table 2.20 presents some of the diseases spread or caused by mites and the associated morbidity and mortality, treatment and prevention. Table 2.21 details control measures for mites.

Table 2.20 **Diseases spread by mites, their treatment and prevention**

Disease	Morbidity and mortality when untreated	Treatment	Prevention
Scabies	Non-fatal but severe cases of infection can lead to eczema	Sulfur ointment or benzyl-benzoate Ivermectin treatment	Good personal and environmental hygiene, adequate supplies of soap and water, frequent bathing and laundry
Scrub typhus	1–60% fatality rates	Antimicrobial Apply disinfecting lotion to skin Disinfect all bed linen and mattresses	Avoid scrub areas or wear protective clothing **or** dust with sulfur powder before going into infected areas

Table 2.21 **The choice of control methods for mites**

Type of mite	Control programme
Trombiculid mite	Treat infected persons Locate infested areas ("mite islands") Destroy the mite by destroying scrub areas or spraying with residual permethrin or deltamethrin insecticide spray around houses, hospitals and camp sites

Ticks

Ticks are fairly rare and are unlikely to be a major hazard in emergency situations. Tick-borne endemic relapsing fever and Lyme disease are the main tick-borne disease that can afflict humans. The use of insecticide impregnated clothing usually provide a very good protection against tick bites.

Fleas

Plague and murine typhus are the two main diseases spread by the flea, both species usually living on rats. Epidemics of plague may occur where there is a high domestic rat population and/or a humid environment at 10–20 °C. The first signs of an epidemic is the occurrence of numerous deaths among domestic rats, followed two weeks later by the first cases of plague among humans. Table 2.22 presents some of the diseases spread or caused by fleas and the associated morbidity and mortality, treatment and prevention. Table 2.23 details control measures for fleas. The flea population must be controlled before the rat population or the fleas will move to humans.

Table 2.22 **Diseases spread by fleas and their treatment and prevention**

Disease	Morbidity and mortality when untreated	Treatment	Prevention
Murine typhus	1–5% fatality rate	Antimicrobial Insecticide dusting powder for the patient, his/her clothing and bedding Airing of bedding	Good personal and environmental hygiene Regular insecticide use Air bedding regularly Dusting and spraying Prevent conditions that attract an increasing rat population
Plague	50–95% case-fatality rate depending on the nutritional status of the population	Antimicrobial – streptomycin Chemoprophylaxis for close contacts Quarantine for patients and contacts	Good personal and environmental hygiene Prevent conditions that attract an increasing rat population Vaccination is only recommended for high-risk groups e.g. health workers and laboratory personnel and not for immediate protection in outbreaks

Table 2.23 **The choice of control methods for fleas**

Type	Control programme
Flea	Baited traps that kill fleas first (insecticide dust) and rats subsequently (anticoagulant)

2.4.2   Vector control strategies

The main methods of arthropod vector control in emergency situations can be classified into the following groups:

- residual spraying,
- personal protection,

- environmental control,
- campsite and shelter design and layout,
- community awareness.

The choice of control strategies in an emergency situation depends on:

- the type of shelter available – permanent housing, tents, plastic sheeting,
- human behaviour – culture, sleeping practices, mobility,
- vector behaviour – biting cycle, indoor or outdoor resting,
- availability of tools, equipment and trained personnel for implementation.

Vector control is strongly recommended in order to reduce incidence of vector borne diseases and prevent outbreaks such as malaria. It is essential that any vector control intervention that is proposed should be planned, implemented in a timely fashion and evaluated by qualified technical personnel. It has to be carried out long enough before the transmission season starts to have the expected impact. The overall vector control interventions should be ready to start as soon as possible.

Recommendations for selecting vector control interventions and insecticides will depend on whether the people to be protected are located in temporary settlements, such as camps, or in permanent communities.

Residual spraying

Residual spraying can be conducted indoors or outdoors. It is important to ensure that:

- the community is involved in planning the spraying exercise and is aware of the conditions required for an effective spraying programme;
- painting or application of fresh mud or mortar is completed prior to the spraying exercise;
- the living accommodation and animal sheds of every household are also sprayed;
- the walls, ceiling and roof are covered with the chemical, paying particular attention to corners and crevices; application should be repeated according to the residual life of the insecticide and the duration of the transmission season.

Indoor residual spraying is a recommended technique for controlling mosquitoes, sandflies and triatomine bugs. It is the most common method in the post-emergency phase when the displaced population is living in more permanent dwellings such as huts or houses. The local mosquito vector must be indoor-resting (at least shortly after blood feeding; seek expert advice) and all houses must be treated, with spraying done just before the beginning of transmission season. It will also help to control bedbugs (which live in walls) and may eventually reduce domestic flea populations. IRS is very effective in almost all epidemiological settings and recommended as the first line intervention to control epidemics. However, implementation is facing growing difficulties (reduced acceptance by populations, lack of trained personnel, high costs) which explain why many programmes are currently shifting to insecticide-treated nets.

Ground space spraying, either ultra-low-volume (ULV) cold mist or thermal fogging, is not the preferred intervention for malaria vector control in emergency situations. It has no residual effect and is not effective against endophilic mosquitoes. In the context of camps, especially in crowded areas, ground space spraying can be resorted to if residual spraying is delayed or cannot be implemented. Treatment must be done either early in the morning or in the evening, before people close the shelters for the night. Applications should be repeated at least once a week. Pyrethrins or pyrethroids are the best choice for such application but organophosphate insecticides are also suitable.

Aerial spraying is not recommended in most emergency situations.

Insecticide resistance

In the context of an emergency, where interventions are planned for limited periods of time until displaced populations can go back home, the selection of insecticide is not a major concern. Pyrethroids used either for residual application, treatment of nets or space spraying are most likely to be effective enough for a few weeks, even if some resistance might occur. However, in some situations, resistance might be high enough to limit the impact of residual applications considerably, especially in the case of non excito-repellent insecticides such as organophosphate and, to a certain extent, carbamates. The situation would be different for longer-term treatments carried out in permanent settlements.

Personal protection

Personal protection against the spread of disease includes a variety of methods: insecticide-treated nets, treated sheets and blankets, personal hygiene, insect repellents and clothing, and dusting powder.

Insecticide-treated nets (ITNs) are primarily used to protect against mosquito bites; however, they also provide a barrier against other vectors such as sandflies, triatomine bugs as well as pests such as bed bugs or cockroaches.

* Non-treated bednets provide partial protection against malaria.
* The effectiveness of bednets can be increased by impregnating them with pyrethroid insecticides.
* The bednets should be soaked in insecticide after every third wash or at least once a year.
* After soaking in the chemical, they should preferably be dried flat so as to maintain an even concentration of the chemical throughout the nets.

ITNs must be available to displaced populations in time to be effective. Distribution of nets must be supplemented by information and educational activities, which may be difficult in an emergency situation. In addition, nets are not easy to hang in tents and are almost impossible to use in shelters. ITNs are regarded more as a tool for long-term prevention, which should be introduced into communities with a number of accompanying measures in order to be effective and sustainable. Free distribution of nets may lead to people refusing to buy nets once they are sold, even at a subsidized price. However, ITNs should be distributed if they are available, especially if house spraying cannot be implemented or has to be delayed. The nets should be treated with insecticide formulations and at dosages recommended by WHO.

Long-lasting insecticidal nets (LLINs) are nets treated at factory level with insecticide either incorporated into or coated around the fibres, resistant to multiple washes and whose biological activity lasts as long as the net itself (3 to 4 years for polyester nets, 4 to 5 years for polyethylene ones).

LLINs offer a practical solution in terms of wash resistance, safe use of coloured nets and purchase of ready-to-use pretreated nets, providing they fulfill specifications. So far, quality control checks carried out by WHO and UNICEF with the two LLINs either recommended or under testing by WHO have shown excellent compliance to specifications on both insecticide treatment and netting specifications.

Advice to control programmes on the purchase and use of LLINs

Be informed of WHO recommendations (regular updates on LLINs or technical information on netting materials and insecticides).

Preferably use WHO-recommended LLINs, especially if difficulties in ensuring proper re-treatment rates are anticipated.

Avoid purchase of factory pretreated nets other than LLINs.

In case LLINs are not available or are not preferred, purchase non-treated nets with insecticide treatment kit(s) bundled.

When and where possible, use ITNs for prevention of several diseases (e.g. malaria + leishmaniasis or lymphatic filariasis).

Check, whenever possible, the quality of nets and insecticides using WHO specifications.

Ensure regular re-treatment of conventional nets already in use, preferably providing treatment free and, once available, use the new long-lasting dipping treatment kits.

Treated sheets and blankets are easy to distribute and effective. In this case, only permethrin (25:75 *cis:trans* isomeric ratio) EC or etofenprox EW should be used, at a dose of 1 g/m². Other pyrethroids are not recommended for this type of application for safety reasons and because of possible skin irritation. Treatment can be made by classical dipping or by spraying sheets and blankets laid on the ground, using either a pressurized hand sprayer or a backpack motorized one. The safety of such treatment is well established, and millions of military uniforms are treated every year with permethrin.

Although shown to be effective in a specific epidemiological situation (Afghanistan), the use of treated sheets and blankets against malaria vectors requires more study in Africa. Since it is always risky to introduce new interventions in emergency situations without previous testing, this intervention is only recommended as a temporary measure or to supplement other well established methods. Insecticide-sprayed tents for "transit" buildings, temporary treatment facilities, and family shelters have not been tested outside Asia. A new technology is under development, based on the incorporation of insecticide into plastic sheeting and tarpaulins used in refugee settings. Instead of being sprayed in situ, insecticide is incorporated within polymer used to produce the plastic sheet and is released over time to the surface of the sheeting. The use of long-lasting insecticide-treated plastic sheeting is promising and undergoing field trials in countries including Angola, Liberia, Pakistan and Sierra Leone.

Personal hygiene. Daily bathing, washing of hands after using the latrine, regular washing of clothes, and good food and water storage practices can prevent the spread of fly-borne diseases.

Insect repellents and clothing. Biting by mosquitoes, flies and ticks can be reduced by wearing long-sleeved shirts and long trousers, and by using insect repellents. Insect repellents can include traditional repellent mixtures, mosquito coils or commercially produced products. These should be used during the biting hours when the species of mosquito is active. Wearing shoes can prevent infestation with jiggers. Permethrin-treated outer clothing worn in the evening or in bed is effective in south Asia but needs testing in highly endemic African conditions.

Dusting powder. Appropriate dusting powders can be used in the treatment of flea and louse infestations. It is important that the powder is applied correctly and that it covers the undergarments and the inner seams of clothing.

Environmental control

Environmental control strategies aim to minimize the spread of disease by reducing the number of vector breeding sites. Some of the most important measures, namely the provision of clean water, the provision and maintenance of sanitary latrines and the efficient and safe disposal of waste, are described earlier in this manual.

Drainage of clean water around water tap stands and rainwater drains is a further important measure in the environmental control of disease vectors. This may include the drainage of ponds, although this may not be acceptable if the water is used for washing

Larvicides destroy the larvae of mosquitoes before they mature into adults. Larvicides may be applied via hand-carried, vehicle-mounted or aerial equipment. The larvicide is added to water at sites that are recognized breeding grounds, such as ponds or water jars, in areas where the breeding sites are limited in number. This is only a temporary solution, however, as larviciding is generally not cost-effective, especially against *An. gambiae*, the main vector in Africa. The multiplicity of *An. gambiae* breeding sites is such that larviciding is almost impracticable. In addition, the efficacy of larvicides is very short (less than a week) and treatment thus requires to be repeated at weekly intervals.

Larviciding can also be used for well-localized and accessible breeding sites of *An. funestus* (permanent swamps with covering vegetation) around camps and residential areas, but as a complement to other methods. In this case, *Bacillus thuringiensis israelensis* (Bti) and temephos (Abate) would be the preferred larvicide. Another problem with larviciding is that, even more than for other interventions, the necessary technical expertise and capacity should be available for planning and implementation.

Longer-term measures, such as land drainage or filling, should be planned and implemented to avoid future spraying.

Campsite and shelter design and layout

Site selection is discussed in detail in Section 2.1.1. It is important to reiterate the importance of avoiding areas that are associated with increased incidence of malaria, onchocerciasis (river blindness), schistosomiasis (bilharziasis), tick fevers and African trypanosomiasis (sleeping sickness).

The following are important aspects of shelter construction.

- Ideally shelters should be of adequate size and spaced sufficiently apart to prevent the spread of communicable diseases.
- The walls should allow residual spraying against biting insects.
- Cracks and crevices should be filled, as they are perfect breeding grounds and habitats for certain vectors.
- Openings in houses should never be sited downwind, as this increases the ability of the vector to reach its host.

Community awareness and health education

Community participation in a vector control programme is essential for its success.

- It allows the implementing agency to develop an awareness of community practices that prevent or encourage the spread of disease.
- Both the community and the vector control team can develop strategies that can be implemented with some degree of success.
- Information on the spread of disease can be disseminated in a culturally sensitive manner.

2.4.3 Rodents and their control

Rodents are disease vectors, reservoir hosts and pests in emergency situations. The main problems associated with rodents are disease transmission, consumption and spoiling of food, damage to stored products, damage to electrical systems, destruction of vegetable gardens, and biting and disturbing people while they sleep (see Table 2.24).

Table 2.24 **Diseases spread by rodents and their treatment and prevention**

Role	Mode of transmission	Disease	Morbidity and mortality when untreated	Treatment	Prevention
As a vector of disease	Rodent urine	Leptospirosis	Low case-fatality rates	Antimicrobial	Rodent-proofing of food stores and containers Good environmental and personal hygiene (e.g. washing of food before eating and storing of cooked food in sealed containers Removal of pools of standing water
	Rodent urine and saliva Food contaminated with rodent body fluids	Lassa fever	15–50% case-fatality rate	Antiviral drug therapy	
	Food contaminated with rodent body fluids	Salmonellosis	2–3% case-fatality among hospital cases	Rehydration Antimicrobial in selected cases	
	Consumption of rodent meat	Toxoplasmosis	Non-fatal but recurrent	Drug therapy	
As a disease reservoir and host to parasite vectors	Fleas and mites – see Section 2.4.1 on diseases				
	Ticks	Tularaemia	Low case-fatality rates	Antimicrobial	
		Rickettsiosis	15–20% case-fatality rate	Antimicrobial	

The elimination of rodents is difficult, particularly in densely crowded camps and in villages or towns, but the rodent population should be kept to a minimum. Rodent control should include safe and regular garbage disposal, trapping, poisoning in selected circumstances, rodent proofing of stores and careful storage of food.

The control of rodents demands an awareness of the behaviour of the types of rodent found in the area. For example, brown rats tend to display neophobia (fear of new objects) and therefore to avoid newly placed traps, bait points, etc. House mice do not show this type of behaviour. *Mastomys* rats (the vectors of Lassa fever) tend to avoid brown and black rats and are therefore not usually found in large numbers in urban environments where the latter are common.

Staff undertaking rodent control programmes must be properly trained and given proper protective clothing.

Public awareness campaigns should be undertaken to inform people on how to control rodents and how to detect evidence of increasing rodent infestation.

Garbage disposal

This is discussed in Section 2.3.

Trapping

- Large numbers of traps should be used.
- There are various types of rodent trap; locally available traps may be more suitable for use by the staff and community than imported equipment.
- The bait must be soft; a banana is ideal for attracting rodents.
- Any rodents caught alive must be killed immediately and carcasses burnt.
- Traps must be checked and reset daily.
- Traps must be placed close to areas where rodents seek food, such as food stores and drains, or next to walls or coverings where they tend to move.
- Traps should be used with care in dwellings. Snap traps have strong springs that can damage children's fingers. The action of certain types of trap (e.g. snap traps) can cause the explosive expulsion of bodily fluids, which can be dangerous in the case of certain diseases (e.g. Lassa fever) that are spread in rodent excreta.

Poisoning

- Poisons must be used only in secure areas, such as stores, since there is a danger of children eating the poison or families eating poisoned rodents to supplement their diet.
- If rodenticides are used, the community must be informed and warned not to consume rodents.
- The best rodenticides are the second-generation anticoagulants (e.g. difenacoum, brodifacoum), which can kill rodents after only a single meal.

Those used should contain Bitrex, which makes the poison too bitter for human consumption.

- Acute poisons such as red phosphorus and cyanide should *never* be used.
- Rodenticides based on pathogens such as *Salmonella* are ineffective and *dangerous* to humans.
- Rodenticides based on reproductive hormones are *not* effective.
- Poisoning programmes should always be preceded by the use of insecticides to treat runs and burrows to kill fleas, which would otherwise leave their rodent hosts and attack humans.
- Poisoning campaigns are not effective on their own in the long term. Other rodent control measures, such as removal of rubbish and improvement of food stores, should always be part of control programmes.
- If rubbish has accumulated and rodent populations have built up, a rodenticide programme should always precede the removal of rubbish, otherwise the rodents will tend to move into dwellings and worsen the health problem.

Making buildings rat-proof

- All doors should be as tight-fitting as possible and should have a galvanized steel strip at least 30 cm deep attached to the bottom to prevent rodent access. Gaps under doors should be reduced to a few millimetres by careful placement of this metal strip.
- All holes in walls should be filled.
- Any drainpipes should be fitted with rat guards.
- Wiring entering buildings should be fitted with rat guards.
- All windows should be covered with 6-mm chicken wire.
- Vegetation should be cleared from around buildings.
- Overhanging vegetation should be removed.
- Stores must have pallets or shelves for storage purposes.
- All opened food must be stored in airtight containers (preferably metal or metal covered).

Food storage guidelines

- All foodstuffs must be stored on pallets or on shelves off the floor at a minimum height of 45 cm to minimize damage by water or rodents. No pallets should be against the wall as this makes cleaning very difficult.
- Pallets should be arranged in stacks not more than four pallets square, with at least 60 cm between stacks to allow access for cleaning.
- Empty sacks must be stored on pallets and not against wall in piles.
- Opened food must be placed in airtight metal bins.

- The store must be well lit and well ventilated.
- The store must be cleaned daily.
- Food in dwellings should be subject to the same careful storage as that in main stores. If possible it should be stored in rodent-proof (metal or well made wooden) bins, which should be inspected regularly for signs of rodent attack.

2.4.4   Monitoring and evaluation of vector control

Successful baseline information has been collected when:
- the vectors prevalent in the area have been identified,
- the types and incidence of disease caused by these vectors have been ascertained,
- the factors that assist in successful reproduction have been identified,
- breeding and resting behaviour of the vector(s) have been identified,
- suitable control measures have been determined.

Some control measures require their implementation by individuals or family units themselves. The indicators for measuring the coverage of such a programme are:
- the percentage of the population that received the relevant information/ education,
- the percentage of the population that implemented the information,
- the percentage reduction or rise in the disease (entomological evaluation can be implemented and analysed only by specialists).

Chemical control measures are usually implemented by specially trained staff. Some indicators of the coverage of such a programme are:
- the percentage of the target area covered with the intervention,
- the supply and safe application of the chemical according to WHO and manufacturer's guidelines,
- the percentage reduction or rise in the vector population.

The major indicators for measuring an effective programme are when:
- suitable control measures are properly implemented and used,
- control measures are successful in reducing incidence of disease (same as above regarding entomological evaluation),
- control measures can be sustained by the population.

2.4.5   Further reading

Equipment for vector control, 3rd ed. Geneva, World Health Organization, 1990.

Kidd H, James JR. *Pesticide index: an index of chemical, common and trade names of pesticides and related crop-protection products*, 2nd ed. Cambridge, Royal Society of Chemistry, 1991.

Thomson MC. *Disease prevention through vector control: guidelines for relief organizations.* Oxford, Oxfam, 1995 (Oxfam Practical Health Guide No. 10).

Vector and pest control in refugee situations. Geneva, Office of the United Nations High Commissioner for Refugees, 1995.

Vector control: methods for use by individuals and communities. Geneva, World Health Organization, 1997.

2.5 Food and nutrition

Food shortages and malnutrition are common features of emergency situations. Ensuring that the food and nutritional needs of an emergency-affected population are met is often the principal component of the humanitarian response to an emergency. When the nutritional needs of a population are not met, this may result in protein–energy malnutrition and micronutrient deficiencies such as iron-deficiency anaemia, pellagra, scurvy and vitamin A deficiency. There is also a marked increase in the incidence of communicable diseases, especially among vulnerable groups such as infants and young children, and these contribute further to the deterioration of their nutritional status.

The objective of this section is to present a brief overview on the nutritional requirements of populations in emergency situations, nutrition interventions, the link between malnutrition and communicable diseases, and the prevention and control of malnutrition.

The nutritional requirements of a population must be assessed to:

- identify the nutritional needs of individuals, families, vulnerable groups and populations as a whole,
- monitor the adequacy of nutritional intake in these groups,
- ensure that adequate quantities of safe food and appropriate food commodities are procured for general rations and selective feeding programmes.

Mean daily per capita requirements are influenced by a number of population and environmental factors, including the following, which should be assessed and taken into account to ensure that energy and protein requirements can be met:

- the age and sex composition of the population,
- mean adult heights and weights (men and women),
- physical activity levels,
- environmental temperatures,
- malnutrition and ill-health,
- food security.

In the acute phase of an emergency, little may be known about the population except the approximate numbers of affected persons. In this situation, an estimated mean daily per capita requirement for a developing country is 2100 kcal$_{th}$[1]. The average safe protein intake per person per day is 46 g from a mixed diet (cereal, pulses and vegetables).

2.5.1   Food requirements

The mean daily per capita energy requirements for some population groups are described in Table 2.25. However, energy requirements will vary depending on the weight, age, gender and physical activity of the individual.

Energy requirements increase during certain specific situations, such as:

- the second and third trimesters of pregnancy,
- lactation,
- infection (e.g. tuberculosis) and recovery from illness (for every 1 °C rise in body temperature there is a 10% increase in energy requirements),
- cold temperatures (an increase of 100 kcal$_{th}$ per person for every 5 °C below 20 °C),
- moderate or heavy labour.

Table 2.25   **Energy requirements for emergency-affected populations in developing countries**

Age (years)	Male (kcal$_{th}$)[a]	Female (kcal$_{th}$)[a]	Male + female (kcal$_{th}$)[a]
0–4	1320	1250	1290
5–9	1980	1730	1860
10–14	2370	2040	2210
15–19	2700	2120	2420
20–59[b]	2460	1990	2230
60+ [b]	2010	1780	1890
Pregnant		285 (extra)	285 (extra)
Lactating		500 (extra)	500 (extra)
Whole population	2250	1910	2080

[a] 1 kcal$_{th}$ = 4.18 kJ
[b] Adult weight: males 60 kg, females 52 kg.
The figures given here for energy requirements are for "light" activity levels. Adjustments need to be made for moderate and heavy activity and environmental temperatures.
Source: The Management of nutrition in major emergencies. Geneva, World Health Organization, 2000.

[1] kcalth = 4.18 kJ

Table 2.26 summarizes the main daily requirements used to calculate the average content of emergency rations.

Table 2.26   **Some important nutritional requirements**

Food type	Quantity
Energy	The mean energy requirement is 2100 kcal$_{th}$ per person per day
Fat/oil	17–20% of the energy should be in the form of edible fats or oils
Protein	10–12% of the energy should be in the form of protein
	Recommended daily protein intake: 46 g from an average mixed diet of cereals, pulses and vegetables

2.5.2   Classification of malnutrition

The impact of food shortages on the health of a population generally becomes apparent through signs of protein–energy malnutrition (PEM), but it should be kept in mind that micronutrient deficiencies are often present as well. In some emergencies, micronutrient deficiencies owing to the poor quality of accessible food items can reach epidemic proportions (e.g. the scurvy epidemic among isolated populations in Afghanistan).

The most reliable indication of *acute* malnutrition is wasting (low weight-for-height) in children aged 6 to 59 months. The severity of PEM in a given individual is thus reflected by the deviation of his/her weight from normal reference weight-for-height values. This can be expressed by either the standard deviation score (Z score), the percentage of the median value, or the percentile.

Calculation of the SD score (Z score) of weight for height:

SD score = (observed value) – (median reference value)/standard deviation of reference population

---

Tables are available (Annex 3) that indicate normalized reference values of weight-for-height together with the corresponding standard deviations, allowing one to calculate the corresponding indices expressing weight-for-height deviations. The presence of symmetrical oedema is another important sign of severe malnutrition.

Stunting or chronic malnutrition (low height-for-age) – comparison of a child's height or length with the reference median height for children of the same age and sex – is of limited value for nutritional screening or assessment surveys in emergencies (except for chronic emergencies and for post-emergency assessments). Stunting indicates a slowing in skeletal growth and, since linear growth responds very slowly compared with weight, it tends to reflect long-standing nutritional inadequacy, repeated infections, and poor overall economic and/or environmental conditions.

Table 2.27 summarizes cut-off values for SD scores, corresponding to standard definitions of moderate and severe malnutrition. The terms "kwashiorkor" and "marasmus" have been omitted to avoid confusion. The clinical syndrome of kwashiorkor includes other features than symmetrical oedema. Severe wasting here corresponds to marasmus (without oedema).

Table 2.27   **Classification of malnutrition**

	Classification	
	Moderate malnutrition	**Severe malnutrition (type)**[a]
Symmetrical oedema	No	Yes (oedematous malnutrition)
Weight-for-height	$-3 \leq$ SD score < -2 [70–79%][b]	SD score < -3 [<70%] (severe wasting)
Height-for-age	$-3 \leq$ SD-score < -2 [85–89%]	SD score < -3 [<85%] (severe stunting)

[a] *The diagnoses are not mutually exclusive.*
[b] *Percentage of the median WHO/National Centre for Health Statistics reference.*

Source: Management of severe malnutrition: a manual for physicians and other senior health workers. Geneva, World Health Organization, 1999.

Measurements of mid-upper arm circumference (MUAC) provide an alternative means of nutritional screening of children between 6 months and 5 years of age. They are useful when resources are limited and where weight and height measurements cannot be made; however, arm circumference measurements can be inaccurate, measuring techniques are difficult to standardize and results can vary widely, both between observers and even with the same observer at different times.

Micronutrient deficiencies in an emergency situation are among the main causes of long-lasting or permanent disability, and most of them are associated with an increased risk of morbidity and mortality. It is useful to distinguish between the deficiencies that are common to many populations particularly in developing countries, such as iron, iodine and vitamin A deficiencies, and those that are specifically seen in *emergencies*, such as thiamine, niacin and vitamin C deficiencies, which must be looked for systematically.

2.5.3   Infection, immunity and nutritional status

The combination of malnutrition and infection causes most of the preventable deaths in emergency situations, particularly among young children. During infection there is an increased need for energy and other nutrients. Malnutrition and micronutrient deficiencies also affect immunity. As a result, people who are malnourished and have compromised immunity are more likely to suffer from diseases such as respiratory infections, tuberculosis, measles and diarrhoeal diseases. Furthermore, in malnourished individuals, episodes of these diseases are more frequent, more severe and prolonged. In addition to the effect of nutrition on disease, the presence of disease leads to further malnutrition, as a result of loss of appetite, fever, diarrhoea and vomiting, which affect nutrient intake and cause malabsorption of nutrients and altered metabolism (see Fig. 2.1). One can conclude that malnutrition is not always simply a consequence of inadequate food supplies but is also linked to repeated infections.

The mechanisms by which malnutrition increases susceptibility to and severity of infection depends on the specific disease. The severity of diarrhoea may be increased in malnourished children because of destruction of the intestinal villi, increased secretion of fluids when pathogens enter the bowel or reduced acidity in the stomach, which prevents the destruction of ingested pathogens. Measles infection damages the immune system and this is exacerbated by vitamin A deficiency. Respiratory infections are thought to have an indirect effect on nutritional status through fever and loss of appetite.

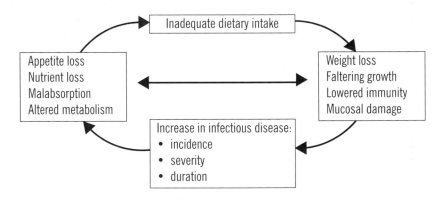

Figure 2.1   **Malnutrition–infection cycle**

Given the strong synergy between nutritional status and morbidity status, and in order to assess and address all the causes of malnutrition in a population, it is important to link nutritional data collected from surveys and nutritional surveillance systems with data on communicable diseases.

2.5.4   Emergency feeding programme strategies

Nutrition interventions: definitions

In emergency situations, the aim should be to ensure that the food needs of the population are met through the **provision of an adequate general ration**. In certain situations, however, there may be a need to provide additional food for a period of time to specific groups who are already malnourished and/or are at risk of becoming malnourished. It must be made very clear that selective feeding is not designed to compensate for the inadequacy of general food rations.

There are two forms of selective feeding programme.

1. Supplementary feeding programmes (SFPs) provide nutritious food in addition to the general ration. They aim to reduce the prevalence of malnutrition and mortality among vulnerable groups and to prevent a deterioration of nutritional status in those most at risk by meeting their additional needs, focusing particularly on young children, pregnant women and nursing mothers.

2. Therapeutic feeding programmes (TFPs) are used to rehabilitate severely malnourished persons. The main aim is to reduce excess mortality. In most emergency situations, the majority of those with severe wasting are infants and young children. There have, however, been cases where large numbers of adolescents and adults have become wasted. In such situations, separate TFP facilities may be established for these groups.

The prevalence of malnutrition is defined as the percentage of the child population (6 months to 5 years of age) who are **below** either the reference median weight-for-height −2SD or 80% of the reference weight-for-height.

Prevalence information is best obtained from conducting a survey (see survey sampling methods in Section 1.4) in children aged 6–59 months (65–100 cm).

Blanket supplementary feeding programmes should be needed only temporarily when prevalence of malnutrition exceeds 15%, or 10% in the presence of other aggravating factors (see footnote to Table 2.28 for a definition of aggravating factors).

Targeted supplementary feeding (i.e. extra food given to selected individuals) is indicated if the prevalence of malnutrition exceeds 10%, or 5% in the presence of other aggravating factors (e.g. high mortality and/or epidemic infectious diseases).

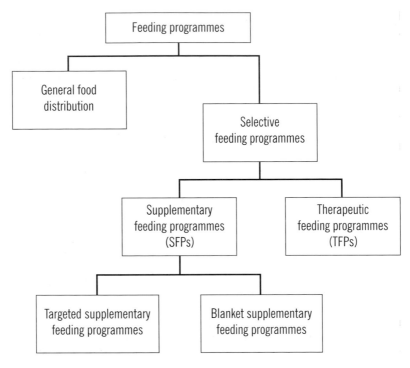

Figure 2.2 **Feeding programme strategy**

Source: *UNHCR/WFP Guidelines for selective feeding programmes in emergency situations.* Geneva, United Nations High Commissioner for Refugees, 1999.

Indications for specific interventions

Table 2.28 provides guidelines for the implementation of selective feeding programmes. The types of selective feeding programme are shown in Table 2.29.

Table 2.28 Decision chart for the implementation of selective feeding programmes[a]

Finding	Action required
Food availability at household level below 2100 kcal per person per day	*Unsatisfactory situation* Improve general rations until local food availability and access can be made adequate
Malnutrition prevalence 15% or more *or* 10–14% with aggravating factors[b]	*Serious situation* • General rations (unless situation is limited to vulnerable groups), plus: – *blanket* supplementary feeding for all members of vulnerable groups especially children and pregnant and lactating women – therapeutic feeding programmes for severely malnourished individuals
Malnutrition prevalence 10–14% *or* 5–9% with aggravating factors[b]	*Risky situation* • No general rations, but: supplementary feeding *targeted* to individuals identified as malnourished in vulnerable groups – therapeutic feeding programmes for severely malnourished individuals
Malnutrition prevalence under 10% with no aggravating factors	*Acceptable situation* • No need for population interventions • Attention for malnourished individuals through regular community services

[a] This chart is for guidance only and should be adapted to local circumstances.
[b] Aggravating factors:
   – general food ration below the mean energy requirement,
   – crude mortality rate more than 1 per 10 000 per day,
   – epidemic of measles or whooping cough,
   – high incidence of respiratory or diarrhoeal diseases.
Source: *The management of nutrition in major emergencies.* Geneva, World Health Organization, 2000.

Table 2.29 **Types of selective feeding programme**

Programme	Objectives	Criteria for selection and target group
Targeted selective feeding programme	Correct moderate malnutrition Prevent the moderately malnourished from becoming severely malnourished Reduce mortality and morbidity risk in children under 5 years Provide nutritional support to selected pregnant and lactating women Provide follow-up services to those discharged from therapeutic feeding programmes	Children under 5 years moderately malnourished Malnourished individuals (based on weight-for-height, MUAC or clinical signs): (1) older children, 5 to 10 years; (2) adolescents; (3) adults and elderly persons; (4) medical referrals Selected pregnant women from date of confirmed pregnancy and nursing mothers until 6 months after delivery, for instance using MUAC < 22 cm as a cut-off indicator for pregnant women Referrals from therapeutic feeding programmes
Blanket selective feeding programme	Prevent deterioration of nutritional situation Reduce prevalence of acute malnutrition in children under 5 years Ensure safety net measures Reduce mortality and morbidity risk	All children under 3 or under 5 years All pregnant women (from date of confirmed pregnancy); nursing mothers (until maximum 6 months after delivery) Other at-risk groups
Therapeutic feeding programme	Provide medical/nutritional treatment for the severely malnourished	Children under 5 years severely malnourished Severely malnourished children older than 5 years, adolescents and adults admitted, based on available weight-for-height standards or presence of oedema Low-birth-weight babies Orphans < 1 year (only when traditional care practices inadequate) Mothers of children younger than one year with breastfeeding failure (only in exceptional cases where relactation through counselling and traditional alternative feeding has failed)

Source: *UNHCR/WFP Guidelines for selective feeding programmes in emergency situations.* Geneva, United Nations High Commissioner for Refugees, 1999.

2.5.5   Food safety: prevention of infection in food preparation

Food is an important vector of pathogens and there is a risk of diarrhoeal disease epidemics when basic food safety principles are not followed. It is estimated that 70% of diarrhoeal episodes in children under the age of 5 years are due to the consumption of contaminated food. There are a number of routine practices that should be adhered to when preparing food, in both the household and in health facilities.

* Ensure an adequate water supply.
* When preparing food or washing utensils, use a chlorinated water supply.
* Store food in sealed containers.
* Ensure that food is covered during cooking and prior to serving.
* Ensure that cooked food is consumed once prepared.
* Cover food when served, if left unattended.
* Place hand-washing facilities outside latrines, living areas and kitchens. Ensure that people use them.
* Ensure an adequate number of sanitary latrines and that they are maintained and used.
* All areas in a feeding centre must be cleaned daily using chlorine as a disinfectant.
* Cover water containers at all times.
* Ensure that water is taken either from a tap or from a clean container.
* Dispose of garbage safely.

2.5.6   Further reading

Caring for the nutritionally vulnerable during emergencies: report of a joint WHO/ UNHCR consultation. Geneva, World Health Organization, 1999 (document WHO/NHD/99.8).

Field guide on rapid nutritional assessment in emergencies. Alexandria, WHO Regional Office for the Eastern Mediterranean, 1995.

Food and nutrition handbook. Rome, World Food Programme, 2000.

Guiding principles for feeding infants and young children during emergencies. Geneva, World Health Organization, 1999 (document WHO/NHD/99.10).

Handbook for emergencies, 2nd ed. Geneva, United Nations High Commissioner for Refugees, 1999.

Management of severe malnutrition: a manual for physicians and other senior health workers. Geneva, World Health Organization, 1999.

The management of nutrition in major emergencies. Geneva, World Health Organization, 2000.

Nutritional guidelines. Paris, Médecins Sans Frontières, 1995.

Pellagra and its prevention and control in major emergencies. Geneva, World Health Organization, 2000 (document WHO/NHD/00.10).

Scurvy and its prevention and control in major emergencies. Geneva, World Health Organization, 1999 (document WHO/NHD/99.11).

Thiamine deficiency and its prevention and control in major emergencies. Geneva, World Health Organization, 1999. (document WHO/NHD/99.13).

UNHCR/WFP Guidelines for selective feeding programmes in emergency situations. Geneva, United Nations High Commissioner for Refugees, 1999.

2.6 Vaccination

The major vaccines used in emergency situations are those against measles, meningococcal meningitis and yellow fever. Measles vaccination is one of the highest priorities in the acute phase of an emergency if vaccine coverage rates in the affected population are below 90%. The main objective of a measles vaccination programme is to prevent an outbreak of measles with the high mortality rates often associated with this disease in emergency situations. In this way, the measles vaccine provides one of the most cost-effective public health tools.

The use of cholera vaccine is recommended only in stable post-emergency situations. Once the acute phase of the emergency is over, plans should also begin to re-establish the Expanded Programme on Immunization (EPI) to routinely immunize children against tetanus, diphtheria, polio and tuberculosis. This should be integrated with the national EPI programme using national vaccination policies, and it is important to involve the national EPI programme from the start of any plan or activity.

The organization of a vaccination campaign requires good management ability and technical knowledge. Responsibilities for each component of the vaccination programme need to be explicitly assigned to agencies and persons by the health coordination agency. The national EPI of the host country should be involved from the outset. National guidelines regarding vaccination should be applied in emergency situations as soon as possible.

2.6.1   Planning and organization of an vaccination campaign

The key steps in the planning of an vaccination campaign are outlined in Table 2.30.

Table 2.30	**Key steps in the planning of an vaccination campaign**

1. **Identify target population**: age group; numbers.

2. **Obtain map of site**: health facilities; roads; access; market places; schools.

3. **Plan vaccination strategies**: mass vaccination campaigns vs. routine vaccination; selective vs. non-selective vaccination.

4. **Define needs**: number of vaccine doses; cold chain equipment; other supplies (auto-destruct syringes, safety boxes, monitoring forms, vaccination cards, tally sheets); staff.

5. **Implement vaccination campaign**: safety of injection; safe disposal of injection material record keeping; individual vaccination cards; other activities (e.g. nutritional supplementation and vitamin A, treatment of complications); health education and social promotion materials.

6. **Evaluate**: coverage percentage vaccinated among estimated target population); incidence of side-effects (post-vaccination surveillance).

Mass vaccination strategies

To implement a mass vaccination campaign in emergencies, there are two main strategies.

1. Vaccination can be carried out at the screening centre on arrival at a camp. This is possible when the screening facility has been set up and the influx of refugees is steady and moderate.

2. Vaccination sites can be set up in different sections of the target area and mass vaccination carried out by outreach teams. This is necessary when the population has already settled at a site or the influx has been too rapid to organize a screening facility.

Routine vaccination strategies

In the case of measles, once the target population has been immunized in the mass campaign, measles vaccination must become part of health care activities. Ongoing vaccination is required to cover:

- children who might have missed the initial vaccination campaign,
- children vaccinated at the age of 6–9 months who must receive a second dose of the vaccine at 9 months,
- new groups of children reaching the age of 6 months.

Vaccination may be **selective**, whereby the vaccination status of the child is checked on the basis of a vaccination card and the vaccine is given if there is no evidence of previous vaccination. In **non-selective** vaccination, vaccination status is not checked and all children are immunized regardless of their immune status. A second dose of measles vaccine has no adverse effect. Non-selective vaccination is preferred in a mass campaign, as it is quicker and leaves little chance for error.

Assessment of risk

The first activity is to assess the need for an vaccination campaign by:

* assessing the risk of an epidemic,
* identifying the size of the population at risk of the disease.

Data on background vaccination coverage in the emergency-affected population should be sought from the Ministry of Health in the country of origin, WHO or UNICEF. If these data are not available, vaccine coverage rates can be assessed by means of a survey using cluster-sampling methodology (see Section 1.4). Perceptions of vaccination can be assessed through focus group discussions with representative groups from the population and/or questions during the vaccination survey.

Assessing logistic requirements

The number of vaccine doses required for a vaccination campaign is 135% of the number in the target population. The same numbers of disposable needles and syringes are also required. These vaccines will require refrigeration until the time of administration; refrigerators and cold boxes are therefore required to maintain the cold chain. Thermometers and temperature monitors are required to ensure the cold chain has been maintained.

The vaccines, cold boxes and thermometers may be available from the Ministry of Health, UNICEF or WHO; alternatively an agency may purchase vaccines and equipment. Syringes and needles will normally also have to be purchased and the cards and registers printed. Advice should be sought from the Ministry of Health, UNICEF or WHO on standard cards and registers, since they may be able to advise on the best printing company and lend registers and cards so that the campaign can be started.

Needs in vaccines

Calculate number of doses based on size of target population, target coverage, proportion of vaccine lost during mass campaign=15%, and reserves to be held=25%.

Total population:		50 000
Target population – e.g. 6 months to 15 years for measles (45% of total):		22 500
[Target population – e.g. 2 to 30 years for meningitis (70% of total):		35 000]
Coverage objective 100%:		22 500
Number of doses to administer :		22 500
Including expected loss of 15%	22 500/85%	26 470
Adding reserve of 25%	26 470 x 125%	33 088
To order:		34 000 doses
If 50 doses per vial, order 680 vials		

Needs in equipment
- **Injection material:**

One sterile needle for one sterile syringe; Sharps containers, trays, kidney dishes depend on number of teams. Incinerators for destruction of used material is essential.

- **Cold chain material:**
- Transport material:

Cool boxes Electrolux type RCW 12 (3000 doses, 14 ice packs) or RCW 25 (7300 doses, 24 ice packs): transport of vaccines, refrigeration 5–7 days

Vaccine carriers (1.7 litres): transport of vaccines, refrigeration 18 hours

Ice packs: keep temperature down in cool boxes, vaccine carriers, vaccination table

- Cold storage equipment:

Refrigerators: storage of vaccines (50 000 doses in 22 litres)

Ice-liners: storage of vaccines when electricity not available 24 hours per day

Freezers: to make ice-packs

- Monitoring equipment:

Thermometers (monitor temperature in each appliance), refrigerator control sheet (monitor temperature in refrigerator, monitoring sheet (indicate temperature of refrigerature)

- **Registration and logistic equipment:**

Vaccination cards (individual), tally sheets. Ropes, tarpaulins, stationery, megaphones

Coordinated and consultative approach

A successful campaign will involve the community, the Ministry of Health, UNICEF, WHO and other international and nongovernmental organizations in the area. It is important to involve all of the stakeholders, as this will ensure that everyone knows the purpose of the campaign, and which people need the vaccine and why. Involvement of the community from the beginning is crucial, and political and traditional leaders should be invited to all major planning meetings. Smaller meetings can subsequently be held with different associations or formal groups within the population, and used to establish suitable times and places for the vaccination campaign. Community health workers can counsel individual families on the importance of the vaccine in question and reassure them about reactions to the vaccine.

Organization of sites

Vaccination sites must be located in such a way as to ensure easy access; additional sites may be required for specific ethnic or other groups. Vaccination campaign sites must be organized so that they are comfortable and operate smoothly. The following are essential points in this respect.

- A waiting area should be provided, with protection against the sun and rain and with seating arrangements and drinking-water. The seating should be organized on a "first come, first served" basis. The person(s) organizing this area can ensure that this principle is maintained, and can also reiterate information on the purpose of the vaccine and possible reactions to the vaccine.

- The entrances and exits must be at different ends of the site.
- A registration point must be placed at the entrance next to the waiting area. Here, the individual's details are entered in the register and he or she is given a card.
- The vaccine administration site is located after the registration point. Two trained health personnel should be allocated to this area, one drawing up the vaccine and the other injecting. There may be more than one vaccine administration team.
- At the exit point, a supervisor must check that the individual has received the card, is registered and has received the vaccine.

Staff training

All staff will need to be trained on the purpose of the vaccination campaign and the technical issues pertinent to the specific vaccine(s). They will also need training on crowd control and communication with the community. The staff involved in the vaccination team will need training on safe injection techniques.

Monitoring coverage

Once the campaign is complete, it is necessary to assess vaccine coverage among the population at risk. This means that every vaccination site and health facility will submit the number of people immunized to a central location. These numbers will be combined to give the total number immunized, and this number will then be divided by the population at risk and multiplied by 100 to provide the percentage of the population covered. These data will help determine if the vaccine campaign is adequate to avert an epidemic, or to prevent further spread if the epidemic has already started.

Coverage can be further validated through a vaccination survey using the EPI 30/7 cluster methodology (see Chapter 1 for details).

2.6.2   Safety of injections

To ensure the safety of injections, WHO and UNICEF have issued a joint policy statement whereby the provision of sufficient quantities of auto-destruct syringes (designed to make reuse impossible) and safety boxes is automatically taken into account, together with high-quality vaccines, in the planning and implementation of all mass vaccination campaigns.

Needles must not be recapped after use, but should be placed immediately into a designated (puncture-resistant) container and disposed of by incineration as soon as possible.

Monitoring injection safety during the campaign

To evaluate injection safety, supervisors must be trained and relevant questions included in their supervisory checklists during implementation and after the campaign.

WHO defines a safe injection as one that:

- does no harm to the recipient,
- does not expose the health worker to avoidable risk,
- does not result in waste that puts other people at risk.

A non-sterile injection is usually caused by:

- reusable syringes that are not properly sterilized before use,
- disposable, one-time-only syringes that are used more than once,
- used syringes and needles that are not disposed of properly.

Unsafe injection practices can result in many complications, the most obvious being abscesses at the site of skin penetration. In most countries, transmission of blood-borne viruses is a less obvious but much more common and serious problem. Hepatitis viruses B and C as well as HIV are the most common and potentially fatal infectious agents that could be transmitted through unsafe injections. Dried blood containing hepatitis B can be infective after one week.

The joint WHO/UNICEF statement states that each injection is to be given with a sterile needle and a sterile syringe, and that single-use needles and syringes must be safely stored and incinerated after use. For all mass campaigns that use an injectable vaccine, auto-destruct syringes and safety boxes (in which needles and syringes can be safely stored pending proper disposal) are recommended. Donors are requested to "bundle" the supplies donated or purchased (i.e. vaccine, auto-destruct syringes and safety boxes).

The person administering the vaccine should practise the following steps to ensure a safe injection:

- Place the patient in a comfortable position; if the patient is a child ensure that the parent/assistant has a firm but not painful grip on the child.
- Ensure that you choose the correct needle for the recipient's age and the injection route.
- Ensure the correct syringe according to dose.
- Ensure that both pieces of equipment are sterile.
- Check the expiry date of the vaccine.
- Ensure that the vaccine is diluted correctly.
- Draw up the correct dose.
- Expel excess air.
- Choose a safe injection site.
- Clean the injection site with an alcohol swab.
- Insert the needle at the correct angle for the recommended injection route.

- Withdraw to ensure you are not in a blood vessel.
- Give the injection slowly.
- Dispose of equipment in a safety box and ensure proper disposal at the end of the vaccination session.

2.6.3   Vaccine storage

There are several types of refrigerator and freezer available, powered by kerosene, electricity, gas and solar energy. The instructions for installation and maintenance that accompany the equipment should be followed. A dial thermometer should be kept in both the refrigerator and the freezer to monitor the temperature, which should be checked and recorded twice daily in a register on the front of the apparatus. If the refrigerator temperature goes below 0 °C or above 8 °C it needs to be readjusted. If the refrigerator breaks down and the cold chain is disrupted, the vaccine in that refrigerator must be discarded as its efficacy can no longer be guaranteed.

The refrigerator must be defrosted regularly. When this is done all vaccines must be placed in a cold box. When vaccines are placed in a cold box for any purpose, a thermometer should be put in the box with them and the temperature monitored. There are two types of cold box available: the small box allows vaccines to be stored for 24 hours, while the larger box stores vaccines safely for up to 7 days.

2.6.4   Measles

Public health importance

Measles remains a major cause of childhood mortality in developing countries. This disease is one of the most serious health problems encountered in emergency situations and has been reported as a leading cause of mortality in children in many recent emergencies. One of the important risk factors for measles transmission is overcrowding. Common complications of measles include malnutrition, diarrhoea and pneumonia; these can all lead to case-fatality ratios of 10–30% among displaced populations.

Measles vaccination

Prevention of measles in emergency situations has two major components: routine vaccination and measles outbreak response. The disease can be prevented by the administration of measles vaccine. Some 95% of individuals vaccinated when over 9 months old gain lifelong immunity.

Mass vaccination is a priority in emergency situations where people are displaced, there is disruption of normal services, there are crowded or insanitary conditions and/or where there is widespread malnutrition, regardless of whether a single case of measles has been reported or not. A measles vaccination campaign should begin as soon as the necessary human resources, vaccine, cold chain equipment and other supplies are available. Measles vaccination should not be delayed until other vaccines become available or until cases of measles have been reported (if cases are reported the campaign should begin within 72 hours of the first report). Vaccination is also a priority in refugee populations from countries with high vaccination rates, as studies have shown that large outbreaks of measles can occur even if vaccine coverage exceeds 80%. It is important to remember that measles is a highly contagious disease requiring 96% coverage for herd immunity to be established.

The presence of several cases of measles in an emergency setting does not preclude a measles vaccination campaign. Even among individuals who have already been exposed and are incubating the natural virus, measles vaccine, if given within 3 days of infection, may provide protection or modify the clinical severity of the illness. If cases of measles occur, isolation is not indicated and children with measles participating in selective feeding programmes should not be withdrawn.

The emergency-affected population must be vaccinated during the first days of the emergency and all new arrivals should be vaccinated. The target age group depends on the vaccine coverage in the country of origin of the affected population. The optimal age group to vaccinate for measles is 6 months through 14 years of age if possible, with a minimum acceptable age range of 6 months through 4 years of age. The target age group for vaccination must be chosen based on vaccine availability, funding, human resources and local measles epidemiology. A measles control plan should be developed and implemented as rapidly as possible while ensuring high quality in coverage, cold chain/logistics, and vaccination safety. Children aged between 6 and 9 months should be revaccinated as soon as they reach 9 months of age.

- Measles vaccination should be accompanied by vitamin A distribution **in children aged 6 months to 5 years** to decrease mortality and prevent complications.

A pre-vaccination count of the target population should be conducted, but this should not delay the start of the vaccination programme. In long-term refugee health programmes, vaccination should be targeted at all children aged between 9 months and 5 years.

If there is insufficient vaccine available to immunize the entire target population, the following high-risk groups should be targeted (in order of priority):

- undernourished or sick children aged 6 months to 12 years who are enrolled in feeding centres or inpatient wards,
- all other children aged 6–23 months,
- all other children aged 24–59 months.

Older children and adults may need to be immunized if surveillance data show that these age groups are being affected during an outbreak. Table 2.31 summarizes the key points concerning measles vaccination and vaccines.

Malnutrition is not a contraindication for measles vaccination; on the contrary, it should be considered a strong indication for vaccination. Similarly, fever, respiratory tract infection and diarrhoea are not contraindications for measles vaccination. Children with HIV infection or clinical AIDS should receive measles vaccine because of the greater risk of severe measles in such cases.

Table 2.31 **Measles vaccination recommendations**

Age	In emergency situations, all children from 6 months to 14 years of age should be immunized, with a minimum age range of 6 months to 4 years if resources are limited. In stable situations, measles vaccine is usually given between 9 and 12 months of age as part of the routine EPI
Dosage	A single dose of 0.5 ml
	If the first dose is given at 6–8 months of age, a second dose must be given at 9 months of age.
	More than one dose can be administered to an individual, as it does no harm and can strengthen immunity; it is a waste of vaccine, however
Route	Subcutaneous injection, usually in the arm, using a new sterile disposable needle (23 gauge) and syringe for each individual
Reactions	Some 5–15% of those vaccinated develop a fever and rash
Side-effects	A small number of cases of encephalitis have been reported
Contraindications	Pregnancy
Instructions for carers	The carer should be told that fever and rash may occur; it should be explained that this is a very mild form of the disease and, unless the temperature is high, there is no need for special action
Records	Each individual should receive a card stating the vaccine given and if a further dose is required
	The name, date of birth, sex and location of each vaccinated individual should be recorded in an appropriate vaccine register
Storage	Measles vaccine is very sensitive to heat and should be stored at a temperature of 2–8 °C (usually on the top shelf of the fridge or in a vaccine carrier)
Reconstitution	Reconstitute with the sterile water that accompanies the vaccine; follow the instructions given on the vial, always check that the vaccine is within its expiry date before reconstitution; unused reconstituted vaccines must be discarded after 8 hours
Storage once reconstituted	The reconstituted vaccine should be placed in the circular hollow of the ice-pack in a shady place

The WHO/UNICEF global measles elimination strategy recommends that a second opportunity for measles revaccination should be offered to all children from 9 months through 14 years, with a minimum interval of one month between the 2 doses.

2.6.5   Meningococcal meningitis

Public health importance

The most common bacterial pathogen causing epidemic meningitis in most countries is the meningococcus, *Neisseria meningitidis*. Meningococcal meningitis is characterized by sudden onset with fever, intense headache, stiff neck, occasional vomiting and irritability. A purpuric rash is a feature of meningococcaemia. Epidemic meningitis has been recognized as serious public health problem for almost 200 years. The main source of the infection is nasopharyngeal carriers. The infection is usually transmitted from person to person in aerosols in crowded places. Rural-to-urban migration and over-crowding in poorly designed and constructed buildings in camps and slums can contribute to transmission. The disease can be treated effectively with appropriate antimicrobial and, with rapid treatment, the case-fatality in an epidemic is usually between 5% and 15%.

Serogroup A and C meningococci are the main causes of epidemic meningitis. In sub-Saharan Africa, serogroup A meningococcal disease is the most common and can lead to periodic, large-scale epidemics during the hot and dry weather in the "meningitis belt". In East Africa, which is outside this belt, the epidemics tend to occur during the cold and dry months. In 2000–2001, serogroup W135 meningococci were identified during outbreaks in Saudi Arabia, and are now spreading in sub-Saharan Africa.

In stable populations, the epidemic threshold is generally an incidence of 15 cases per 100 000 inhabitants per week, in 1 week if the population is greater than 30 000, and 5 cases in 1 week *or* doubling of the number of cases over a 3-week period if the population is less than 30 000. When the epidemic threshold is reached, a mass vaccination campaign should be implemented in the at-risk population (for more details see Section 4.2.2).

In emergency-affected populations, however, particularly in overcrowded situations, the threshold for action is lower and the decision to implement a vaccination campaign must be taken locally in consultation with the relevant authorities, such as WHO or the Ministry of Health. Microbiological confirmation should be sought as a matter of urgency, but this should not delay the start of a vaccination campaign.

Meningitis vaccine

Meningococcal meningitis A and C can be prevented by vaccination. The vaccine is effective within 8–14 days. Some 90% of recipients over 18–24 months of age seroconvert and are protected against the disease. Vaccine-induced immunity lasts about 5 years in adults and older children, while younger children are protected for approximately 2 years. A quadrivalent vaccine is also available for combined vaccination against serogroups A, C, Y and W135. Vaccination recommendations for meningococcal meningitis are summarized in Table 2.32.

Table 2.32　**Meningococcal meningitis vaccination recommendations**

Age	The group at highest risk of meningococcal meningitis is children aged 2–10 years; this should be the priority group during vaccination campaigns
Dosage	A single dose of 0.5 ml
Route	Deep subcutaneous or deep intramuscular, using a new sterile disposable needle and syringe for each individual; mixing the meningitis vaccine in the same vial or syringe as live virus vaccines, such as measles, is not recommended
Side effects	Up to 71% of the recipients will develop a mild local reaction at the injection site; with current, highly purified vaccine preparations, fever is seen in less than 2% of vaccinees
Contraindications	Febrile illness, known hypersensitivity, pregnancy
Instructions for carers or recipients	The carer/recipient should be told to expect a fever and swelling around the injection site; it should be explained that this is a very mild form of the disease, but if the fever is high they should give paracetamol and return to the doctor
Records	Ensure that the individual is given a record of the vaccine and also that the vaccinators retain a record in a register
Storage	Store at 2–8 °C; do not allow the vaccine to freeze
Reconstitution	There is a specific diluent with each vial of vaccine, and this is the only diluent to be used with the vaccine; read the vial and follow the instructions given, always check that the vaccine is within its expiry date before reconstitution
Storage once reconstituted	Unused vaccine should be disposed of within 1 hour of reconstitution

2.6.6　Yellow fever

Public health importance

Yellow fever is a viral disease transmitted by mosquitoes and occurs primarily in Africa and South America. There is no specific treatment, but supportive therapy for patients should be provided. The overall case-fatality rate is less than 5%, although the rate among patients with jaundice is 20–50%.

Yellow fever vaccine

Vaccination is the primary means of preventing yellow fever. The yellow fever vaccine offers a high level of protection, with seroconversion rates of 95% or higher for both adults and children. The duration of immunity is at least 10 years and probably lifelong. The serological response to yellow fever vaccine is not inhibited by simultaneous administration of BCG, diphtheria, pertussis, tetanus, measles and poliomyelitis vaccines. Reactions to yellow fever vaccine are generally mild. It can be given to asymptomatic patients infected with HIV, but should not be given to symptomatic HIV-infected persons or other immuno-suppressed individuals. For theoretical reasons, yellow fever vaccine is not routinely recommended for pregnant women; however, there is no evidence that vaccination of a pregnant woman is associated with abnormal effects on the fetus. In an outbreak, the risk of disease would outweigh the small theoretical risk to the fetus from vaccination. Recommendations regarding yellow fever vaccination are summarized in Table 2.33.

Table 2.33 **Yellow fever vaccination recommendations**

Age	All individuals over 6 months of age and the members of a high-risk population should receive the vaccine; in some countries the vaccine is part of the national EPI programme and is given at the same time as measles vaccine
Dosage	A single dose of 0.5 ml
Route	Deep subcutaneous injection using a new sterile disposable needle (23 gauge) and syringe for each individual
Side effects	Some 5% of individuals develop a low-grade fever, headache or myalgia within the first 10 days after vaccination
	Immediate hypersensitivity reactions with rash, urticaria or asthma occur in less than 1 per million individuals and usually among those with known egg allergy
	Serious adverse reactions are extremely rare: 22 cases of encephalitis have been reported to WHO since 1945, in relation to over 200 million doses of 17D yellow fever vaccine given worldwide. Most of those affected were children under 4 months of age
Contraindications	Children under 6 months of age, pregnancy, and symptomatic HIV-infected persons or other immunosuppressed individuals
Instructions for carers or recipients	The individual should be told that a low-grade fever, headache or myalgia may occur within the first 10 days after vaccination, and that if any other condition develops they should seek medical attention
Records	Each individual should receive a certificate as a record of vaccination; each individual's name should be recorded in an appropriate vaccine register
Storage	Live attenuated 17D yellow fever vaccine is heat-sensitive, and should be transported and stored either frozen or at a temperature of 4–8 °C
Reconstitution	Reconstitute with the diluent that accompanies the vaccine; follow the instructions given on the vial; always check that the vaccine is within its expiry date prior to reconstitution
Storage once reconstituted	Reconstituted vaccine is very unstable and should ideally be discarded within 1 hour, although it can last for 6 hours if kept cool

2.6.7 Oral cholera vaccines

New generation orally administered cholera vaccines (OCV) have passed the stage of research and development and two formulas are commercially available. Currently, the main users of marketed OCV have been individual travelers from industrialized countries who expect to be exposed temporarily to the risk of cholera while traveling in endemic areas. Recently, there has been renewed interest in using oral cholera vaccines in mass vaccination campaigns, in conjunction with traditionally recommended control measures such as provision of safe water and improved sanitation.

Several mass-vaccination campaigns using OCV have been performed with the support of WHO. In 2000, the Federated States of Micronesia exposed to an ongoing outbreak in Pohnpei Island decided on using the live-attenuated oral cholera vaccine CVD 103-HgR to limit the spread of the outbreak. A retrospective analysis suggested that mass vaccination with OCVs can be a useful adjunct tool for controlling outbreaks, particularly if implemented early and in association with other standard control measures. Further, campaigns using the recombinant killed whole cell oral cholera vaccine rBS-WC have been conducted in Mozambique (2003/2004), Darfur (2004) and Sumatra (2005) to protect at risk populations from potential cholera outbreaks. The experience gained as a result from those interventions is encouraging. Big challenges however remain with regard to risk assessment, identification of the target population and logistics among others.

Currently, OCVs may prove useful in the stable phase of emergencies as well as in endemic settings especially when given pre-emptively. Available data indicates that current OCV are safe and offer good protection for an acceptable period of time. The use of OCV should be through well designed demonstration projects and should be complementary to existing cholera control strategies. These demonstration projects should result in gaining evidence on when best to use OCVs as an additional public health tool.

Traditional injectable cholera vaccines are considered insufficiently protective and too reactogenic. Their use has never been recommended by WHO.

2.6.8 Further reading

WHO-UNICEF policy statement for mass immunization campaigns. Geneva, World Health Organization, 1997 (document WHO/EPI/LHIS/97.04).

Measles

Conduite à tenir en cas d'épidémie de rougeole [Management of measles epidemics]. Paris, Médecins Sans Frontières, 1996.

Toole MJ et al. Measles prevention and control in emergency settings. *Bulletin of the World Health Organization*, 1989, **67**:381–388.

WHO-UNICEF joint statement on Reducing measles mortality in emergencies World Health Organization, 2004 (document WHO/V&B/04.3).

Epidemic meningitis

Management of epidemic of meningococcal meningitis. Paris, Médecins Sans Frontières, 2004.

Control of epidemic meningococcal disease: WHO practical guidelines, 2nd ed. Geneva, World Health Organization, 1998 (document WHO/EMC/BAC/98.3).

Detecting meningococcal meningitis epidemics in highly endemic African countries: WHO recommendation. *Weekly Epidemiological Record*, 2000, **75**(38):306–309.

Yellow fever

Adverse events following yellow fever vaccination. *Weekly Epidemiological Record*, 2001, **76**:217–218.

District guidelines for yellow fever surveillance. Geneva, World Health Organization, 1998 (document WHO/EPI/GEN/98.09).

Robertson SE. *The immunological basis for vaccination. Module 8: yellow fever*. Geneva, World Health Organization, 1993 (document WHO/EPI/GEN/93.18).

Robertson SE et al. Yellow fever: a decade of re-emergence. *Journal of the American Medical Association*, 1996, **276**:1157–1162.

Silva J et al. *Vaccine safety: yellow fever vaccine. Report of the Technical Advisory Group on Vaccine Preventable Disease*. Washington, DC, Pan American Health Organization, 2000.

Yellow fever –Technical Consensus Meeting, Geneva, 2–3 March 1998. Geneva, World Health Organization, 1998 (document WHO/EPI/GEN/98.08).

Oral cholera vaccines

Potential use of oral cholera vaccines in emergency situations. Report of a WHO meeting, Geneva, Switzerland, 12–13 May 1999. Geneva, World Health Organization, 1999 (document WHO/CDS/CSR/EDC/99.4 – www.who.int/topics/publications).

Cholera vaccines: A new public health tool? Report, 10–11 December 2002, Geneva, Switzerland; WHO/CDS/CPE/ZFK/2004.5 (www.who.int/topics/publications).

Cholera vaccines: Published on 20 April 2001, Vol. 76, **16**:117–124 (www.who.int/vaccines-documents/PP-WER/wer7616.pdf).

Calain P et al. Can oral cholera vaccination play a role in controlling a cholera outbreak? *Vaccine*, 2004, **22**:2444-2451.

Lucas ME et al. Effectiveness of mass oral cholera vaccination in Beira, Mozambique. *New England Journal of Medicine*, 24 Feb. 2005; **352(8)**:757–767.

Update on cholera vaccines. *Weekly epidemiological record*, 2005, **80**(31):265–268.

2.7 Health education and community participation

Health education and community participation in interventions play a key role in communicable disease prevention and control.

Some areas where health education and community participation can be beneficial:

• Improving recognition of severe disease by the population.
• Improving health-seeking behaviour.
• Promotion of early and appropriate use of ORS in treatment of diarrhoeal disease.
• Promotion of vector control programmes e.g. use of ITNs.
• Promotion of hygiene/hand-washing for prevention of diarrhoeal disease.
• Promotion of safe water use and storage.
• Promotion of appropriate sanitation.
• Promotion of environment management to prevent degradation and vector reproduction.
• Active case-finding in outbreaks.
• Communicable disease surveillance system.
• Data collection for mortality and population statistics.
• Community mobilization for vaccination campaigns/vaccination.

Principles of effective community participation in emergencies:

• Have knowledge of displaced or refugee, and host population communities:
  – social structure,
  – vulnerable groups,
  – members of formal organizations,
  – members of semi-formal organizations such as schools, faith-based organizations, social organizations,
  – community leaders or spokespeople,
  – family/kin networks,
  – roles within community,
  – customs and practices, e.g. belief against giving water to sick children (use of colouring to make water look like medicine to render it culturally acceptable), use of chaddars as top-sheets for sleeping (can impregnate with permethrin for prevention of mosquito bites).
• Identify community concerns and priorities.
• Use community members to collect data.
• Involve community in implementation of activities, e.g. surveillance of deaths, case-finding, health education, sanitation and environmental improvement.
• Ensure effective communication between population, host communities, government and agencies involved in response.

Volunteer collaboration

Volunteer collaboration within a community enables participatory mapping of priorities and needs, allows working with elders and leaders for advocacy and support, identifies volunteers who can help in organizing the community to address problems, and enables reporting information to the coordination body or local district. Success depends on whether volunteers' actions are measurable and make a difference. Important questions to ask include: Are there volunteers in each community? Are there enough volunteers to cover the whole community? Do the volunteers know the community and how to approach health topics? Do the volunteers know key messages for each health problem? Do the volunteers know what information to collect in order to measure effectiveness?

Volunteers should be from the community in which they work, even in emergencies. They should work with their elders, leaders and local health staff (health workers and traditional birth attendants). Volunteers should know the traditional beliefs about diseases and know what priority health problems the community wants to solve. They should also know what other groups are doing in their community about priority health problems and know the families and visit them regularly to provide key messages.

Volunteers are part-time and need to reorganize themselves in order to accomplish their designated tasks. Community action where groups of volunteers work at the same time on a project requires a leader to ensure coordination.

3. SURVEILLANCE

This chapter outlines the key steps in setting up and running a surveillance system in an emergency.

3.1 General principles

Surveillance is the ongoing systematic collection, analysis and interpretation of data in order to plan, implement and evaluate public health interventions.

A surveillance system should be simple, flexible, acceptable and situation-specific. It should be established at the beginning of public health activities set up in response to an emergency.

Public health surveillance classically comprises six core activities (detection, registration, confirmation, reporting, analysis and feedback) that are made possible through four support activities (communication, training, supervision and resource provision).

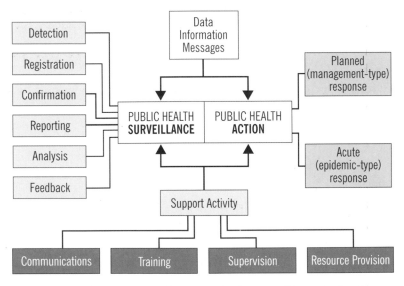

Figure 3.1   **Conceptual framework of public health surveillance and action**

If systematic surveillance activities are not possible, for example due to lack of access, an alternative means of monitoring specific health-related trends is to sample the population through repeated health surveys, using design and questionnaires similar to those used for the initial rapid assessment (see Chapter 1).

3.2 Objectives

The objectives of a surveillance system in an emergency are to:

- identify public health priorities;
- monitor the severity of an emergency by collecting and analysing mortality and morbidity data;
- detect outbreaks and monitor response;
- monitor trends in incidence and case-fatality from major diseases;
- monitor the impact of specific health interventions (e.g. a reduction in malaria incidence rates after the implementation of vector control programmes);
- provide information to the Ministry of Health, agency headquarters and donors to assist in health programme planning, implementation and adaptation, and resource mobilization.

DATA	→	INFORMATION	→	ACTION
Number of deaths		Crude mortality rate		Mortality reduction measures

Before starting to design a surveillance system, the following questions should be asked:

- What is the population under surveillance: displaced population, local population?
- What data should be collected and for what purpose?
- Who will provide the data?
- What is the period of time of the data collection?
- How will the data be transferred (data flow)?
- Who will analyse the data and how often?
- How will reports be disseminated and how often?

3.3 Setting surveillance priorities

It is not possible to monitor everything in an emergency. At field level, the health coordination team must identify a limited number of priority diseases that pose a threat to the health of the population. This selection process must be done at the beginning of health care activities in an emergency.

The choice of surveillance priorities should answer the following questions:

- Does the condition result in a high disease impact (morbidity, disability, mortality)?
- Does it have a significant epidemic potential (e.g. cholera, meningitis, measles)?
- Is it a specific target of a national, regional or international control programme?
- Will the information to be collected lead to significant and cost-effective public health action?

Experience from many emergency situations has shown that certain diseases/ syndromes must always be considered as priorities and monitored systematically. In the acute phase of an emergency, the major diseases/syndromes that should be reported are:

- bloody diarrhoea,
- acute watery diarrhoea,
- suspected cholera,
- lower respiratory tract infection,
- measles,
- meningitis.

In certain geographical areas, other diseases that are endemic or that represent an epidemic threat, such as malaria or viral haemorrhagic fevers may have to be included.

In the post-emergency phase, additional diseases that should be reported include:

- tuberculosis,
- HIV/AIDS,
- neonatal tetanus,
- sexually transmitted infections.

See Annex 5 for case definitions for each disease/syndrome.

When setting up surveillance systems, it is important to be aware of health conditions that have local distribution and include these in the surveillance programme. In parts of West Africa, for example, Lassa fever should be included in the list of priority diseases for surveillance. In areas where typhus has caused problems in the past, routine surveillance should include reporting both of suspected/confirmed cases of the condition and of infestations with body lice, the vector of the disease.

In addition, other health events of importance, e.g. injuries, wound infections may need to be added to the list of surveillance priorities.

3.4 Data collection methods

There are three main methods for collecting data in emergency situations: routine reporting (including epidemic-prone diseases requiring immediate notification), surveys and outbreak investigations (see Table 3.1).

Table 3.1 **Data collection methods**

Method	Indication	Frequency
Routine reporting: endemic	Routine surveillance	Weekly (emergency phase), then monthly
Alert system: epidemic (early warning)	Epidemic-prone diseases	Immediate notification
Outbreak investigations	Declared outbreaks	Ad hoc
Surveys	Delays in setting up routine surveillance, or Household-based data (e.g. nutrition, basic needs, vaccination)	Depends on specific needs or questions addressed

In routine reporting, clinical workers collect data on the number of cases and deaths from priority diseases. Data are reported as part of the day-to-day work of the hospital, health clinic or outreach post. Routine data are usually recorded in an inpatient or outpatient register, and are then transferred to summary tally sheets at the end of each week. At the end of the reporting period, the information is sent to the health coordinator for compilation and analysis. Case definitions for epidemic-prone diseases listed in the surveillance system should include specific indications on when immediate notification is mandatory: either as soon as a single case is suspected (e.g. haemorrhagic fevers, measles, yellow fever) or after an indicated alert threshold is reached (e.g. epidemic meningitis).

Surveys aim at collecting data on a representative sample of the emergency-affected population (or of a defined subgroup). When the organization of a sustainable surveillance system has to be delayed, iterative surveys can provide the information needed for emergency decisions. Survey principles and methods are described in Chapter 1.

Outbreaks entail active case-finding and in-depth investigation, whereby attempts are made to identify the cause of an unusual number of cases of death or disease and to implement control measures. These investigations are dealt with in Chapter 4.

3.5 Case definitions

Case definitions must be developed for each health event/disease/syndrome. Standard WHO case definitions are given in Annex 5, but these may have to be adapted according to the local situation. If possible, the case definitions of the host country's Ministry of Health should be used if they are available. What is important is that all of those reporting to the surveillance system, regardless of affiliation, use the same case definitions so that there is consistency in reporting.

Case definitions considered here are designed for surveillance purposes only. A surveillance case definition is not to be used for the management of patients and is not an indication of intention to treat.

In many emergency situations, where there is no timely laboratory access for confirmation of certain diseases (e.g. cholera), public health action can be based on a presumptive diagnosis. Surveillance case definitions should indicate, if appropriate, when a case is suspect, probable or confirmed.

Table 3.2 **Case classification**

Type of case	Criteria
Suspected case	Clinical signs and symptoms compatible with the disease in question but no laboratory evidence of infection (negative, pending or not possible)
	Example for meningococcal meningitis: suspected case = meets clinical case definition
Probable case	Compatible clinical signs and symptoms, *and* additional epidemiological (e.g. contact with a confirmed case) or laboratory (e.g. screening test) evidence for the disease in question
	For meningococcal meningitis: probable case = suspected case + turbid CSF or ongoing epidemic or epidemiological link to confirmed case
Confirmed case	Definite laboratory evidence of current or recent infection, *whether or not* clinical signs or symptoms are or have been present
	For meningococcal meningitis: confirmed case = suspected or probable case + laboratory confirmation
	Note that in outbreaks of certain diseases, clinical symptoms are not present in a proportion of people, however they are counted as confirmed cases with laboratory evidence since subclinical infection is a major source of transmission

Some infectious diseases, such as neonatal tetanus, normally do not require laboratory confirmation and can be reported on the basis of pure clinical criteria. Others, such as pulmonary tuberculosis, need to be confirmed by laboratory tests before official reporting of a case. In other instances, disease presentation can correspond to various or multiple causative organisms (e.g. sexually-transmitted infections) and the demonstration of the etiologic agent(s) is irrelevant for adequate case management or public health action. In such cases, a "syndromic" case definition is adequate. Presumptive (suspect or probable) or syndromic case definitions may assist the Outbreak Control Team in establishing the likely occurrence of an outbreak and in taking appropriate control measures, before laboratory results become available.

Case definitions may have to be adapted to the circumstances, as illustrated by the following two classic examples.

✔ The case definition recommended by WHO for suspected cholera varies, depending on cases being seen during a confirmed outbreak or not (see Annex 5).

✔ For malaria, a clinical case definition may need to suffice during the acute phase of an emergency since microscopy confirmation of all suspected cases may be difficult, particularly in high-transmission areas where the case-load is large*. In unstable endemic areas, even the best clinical algorithms may wrongly classify a disease episode as being malaria and may also fail to identify many true cases of malaria; diagnosis by microscopy or RDTs should be provided as soon as possible to improve case management and surveillance. In stable high-transmission areas, where a high proportion of the population can have parasitacmia without symptoms, microscopy may not be so useful for the definition of cases; anaemia in children and pregnant women, low birth weight and high rates of splenomegaly (although not very specific) may serve as supporting indicators.

3.6 Minimum data elements

Through appropriate data collection methods (see Section 3.4), the surveillance system must capture at least the following categories of health-related parameters:

– mortality,
– morbidity,
– population figures and trends (demographic data),
– nutrition,
– basic needs,
– programme activities (including vaccination).

For each category, key indicators must be calculated to allow analysis of trends and comparison of the data. Ideally, mortality and morbidity data should be reported as the incidence for a given size of population, so demographic data are needed to calculate them (e.g. incidence of malaria per 1000 population per month).

If the population denominators are not taken into account, or demographic changes are not monitored, simple changes in numbers of cases of a disease/

---

* However, increasing availability of rapid diagnostic tests (RDTs) for falciparum malaria may allow confirmation of malaria cases.

syndrome can be highly misleading in terms of assessment of potential epidemics, since they may represent changes in the numbers of the targeted population rather than changes in incidence. Nevertheless, case numbers should be collected and reported (with suitable disclaimers as to accuracy) even in the absence of demographic data. Even if the increased numbers of cases of a disease are not indicative of an outbreak, they nevertheless present medical staff and logistic services with an increased demand that must be quantified and met.

Malnutrition and compromised access to basic needs are frequently seen in emergencies and have a major impact on disease susceptibility. Available data (preferably from household surveys) on malnutrition, basic household needs and vaccination coverage should be collected as well, and included in the periodical analysis of surveillance data, together with communicable diseases. Sample household survey forms are included in Annex 2.

3.6.1 Mortality

The crude mortality rate (CMR) is the most important indicator in an emergency, as it indicates the severity and allows monitoring of the evolution of an emergency. In most developing countries, the average crude mortality rate is about 18 deaths per 1000 population per year, i.e. 0.5 per 10 000 per day. Early in an emergency, mortality is expressed in deaths per 10 000 people per day. The acute phase of an emergency is defined as when the CMR goes above 1 per 10 000 per day in a displaced population (see Table 3.10).

Crude mortality rate is the total number of deaths in the population (over 1 week or 1 month), divided by the average population at risk during that time (week/month), multiplied by 1000 (this gives number of deaths per 1000 per time frame chosen). This can then be converted to deaths per 10 000 per day.

• On causes of death:

Proportionate mortality: Proportionate mortality describes the proportion of deaths in a specified population over a period of time attributable to different causes. Each cause is expressed as a percentage of all deaths, and the sum of the causes must add to 100%. These proportions are not mortality rates, since the denominator is all deaths, not just the population in which the deaths occurred. For a specified population over a specified period: Proportionate mortality = [deaths due to a particular cause / deaths from all causes] x 100

Cause-specific mortality rate: The cause-specific mortality rate is the mortality rate from a specified cause for a population. The numerator is the number of deaths attributed to a specific cause. The denominator is the at-risk population size at the midpoint of the time period.

3.6.2 Morbidity

Priority diseases/syndromes will have been selected by the health coordination team depending on the main disease threats in the emergency area. For maximum efficiency, it is important to limit the number of diseases reported and the data collected for each case. Health facilities are generally the main source of morbidity data in an emergency. Where access to or use of health facilities is limited, such data might not be representative of the condition of the overall population. For certain epidemic-prone diseases, however, it is essential that all cases are detected in the community and reported. Social mobilization by community workers may be useful in the acute phase of an emergency to ensure that those among the emergency-affected population that are ill access to health care services.

The **incidence** is the number of new cases of a specified diseases reported over a given period. The number of new cases reported should be counted (over 1 week/month), divided by the average population at risk during that time (mid-week/month), and multiplied by 1000 (or any other global number to allow easy interpretation). The incidence is then specified as number of new cases per 1000 people (or the number that you have multiplied by).

Case-fatality rate (CFR): the percentage of persons diagnosed as having a specified disease who die as a result of that disease within a given period, usually expressed as a percentage (cases per 100).

Attack rate (outbreaks): The cumulative incidence of cases (persons meeting case definition since onset of outbreak) in a group observed over a period during an outbreak.

3.6.3 Population figures and trends

Demographic data deal with the size and composition of the population affected by an emergency. They are needed to calculate:

• the size of the population targeted for humanitarian assistance,

• the size of high-risk groups (e.g. under-fives),

• the denominators for mortality, morbidity and other rates,

• the resource needs for health interventions.

In most emergencies, demographic data can be obtained from public institutions or United Nations agencies. It is important that all agencies working in an emergency agree on and use the same population figures. In certain emergency situations involving displaced persons, the local population in the affected area should also be included in the total population. The demographic data that need to be collected are given in Table 3.3.

Table 3.3   Demographic data to be collected

- Total population size

- Population under 5 years of age

- Numbers of arrivals and departures per week

- Predicted number of future arrivals (if available)

- Place of origin

- Number of people in vulnerable groups, such as unaccompanied children, single women, pregnant women, woman-headed households, destitute elderly people and people with disabilities

Table 3.4 gives the standard age distribution in developing countries. However, the age structure of displaced populations is often heavily distorted, with excess numbers of children, women and the elderly. Young males of military age are often under-represented.

Table 3.4   Standard age distribution in developing countries

Age group	Proportion of total population
0–4 years	17%
5–14 years	28%
15+ years	55%
Total	**100%**
Women 15–44 years	20%

3.6.4   Basic needs

Basic needs in emergencies are listed in Annex 1 (see also nutritional require-ments in Section 2.5.1).

While questionnaires can be easily administered on convenience samples of the population visiting health facilities, results of such surveys are biased and do not represent the basic needs of the whole population. Basic needs are better addressed through household-based surveys, using the same techniques as those used for the initial rapid survey.

3.6.5   Nutrition

Data from paediatric centres or malnutrition clinics are important in monitoring the performance of health-centre-based programmes, but they do not represent the nutritional status of the whole population affected by the emergency. As with basic needs, malnutrition should be assessed at household level if relevant community-based actions have to be planned.

3.6.6 Programme activities, including routine vaccination

Monitoring activities at all levels of the health system set up in emergencies is an integral part of surveillance. Typical activities to be registered include: number of vaccinations, number of consultations, number of admissions, and number of children in supplementary or therapeutic feeding programmes.

3.6.7 Post-emergency phase

As the emergency evolves from the acute to a more chronic phase, the minimal surveillance system initially put in place has to expand. Useful adaptations can include:

- more detailed data: indices by sex, high risk groups,
- better quality of data,
- updating denominators,
- capturing more events (e.g. reproductive health, child health, HIV; tuberculosis, sexually transmitted infections).

3.7 Data sources for routine surveillance

The six categories of data are collected from the sources given in Table 3.5.

Table 3.5 **Categories and sources of data**

Categories	Sources
Mortality	Health facilities, home visitors, grave-watchers, numbers of shrouds issued, community leaders
Morbidity	Health facilities, home visitors
Demography	Local health and administrative services, other agencies
Basic needs	Agencies involved in water/sanitation, food distribution
Nutrition	Nutritional surveys, food distribution agencies
Programme activities, including vaccination	Health facilities, EPI programme

The main sources of data for routine surveillance are clinic registers used for day-to-day activity in health facilities. Recording the number and causes of death in an emergency can be difficult, as many deaths may take place outside the health facility. Home visitors can play an important role in collecting information on numbers and causes of deaths, using a "verbal autopsy" method with the family of the deceased person.

Data on demography and basic needs will usually be available from specialized agencies, such as UNHCR and nongovernmental organizations providing rehabilitation of water and sanitation facilities.

A standard form should be developed for clinical workers to compile the data at the end of each week (sample weekly morbidity and mortality forms are provided in Annex 4). These forms should be simple, and clear, have enough space to write information clearly and ask only for information that will be used. The minimum data needed for each health event/disease under routine surveillance include:

- case-based data for reporting and investigation: name, date of birth (or age, approximate if necessary if date of birth is not known), camp district/area, date of onset, treatment given (Yes/No) and outcome; this is not necessary for all events and often a tally may suffice as, in a major emergency, health personnel will not have the time to record case-based information;

- aggregated data for reporting: number of cases (less than 5 years old, 5 years old and over) and number of deaths.

Outbreak alert forms should also be available for clinical workers for immediate reporting of a disease of epidemic potential (Annex 6).

It is important in filling out the forms that clinical workers:

- record the exit diagnosis (based on agreed case definitions);

- avoid double counting – if a patient comes to the health centre for a follow-up visit for the same condition , he/she should be counted only once;

- only count those cases diagnosed by a professional health worker, unless well motivated community workers trained in specific programme areas can be identified as reliable sources of information (e.g. for the poliomyelitis eradication programme).

The system should include **zero reporting**. Each site should report for each reporting period, even if it means reporting zero cases. This avoids the confusion of equating "no report" with "no cases".

Sources of mortality, morbidity and demographic data are given in Tables 3.6–3.8.

Table 3.6   **Sources of mortality data**

Health facilities

Hospital/health facility death records – inpatient registers/outpatient registers

Home visitors/community workers

Grave-watchers trained to provide 24-hour coverage on a designated single burial site and report on the daily number of burials

Home visitors trained to use the verbal autopsy method for expected causes of death with standard forms

Religious/community leaders

Community workers trained to report deaths for a defined section of the population, e.g. 50 families

Other agencies

Records of organizations responsible for burial

Agencies distributing shrouds free of charge to families of the deceased to encourage reporting of deaths

Table 3.7   **Sources of morbidity data**

Health care facility records: outpatient department (OPD)and inpatient department (IPD) registers and records in camp clinics, hospitals, feeding centres and local communities

Health workers and midwives within the displaced population

Table 3.8   **Sources of demographic data**

Registration records maintained by camp administrators, local government officials, United Nations agencies, religious leaders, etc.

Mapping

Aerial photographs or global positioning systems

Census data

Interviews with community leaders among the displaced population

Cross-sectional surveys

3.8   Identifying tasks and responsible persons

The surveillance team must include a health coordinator, clinical workers, community workers, a water and sanitation specialist and representatives of local authorities. The health coordinator is usually the team leader. The team should meet at least daily in the acute phase of the emergency and weekly or monthly when the situation stabilizes.

One of the most important requirements for a good surveillance system is a network of motivated clinical workers trained in case detection and reporting.

These clinical workers will have many other duties, primarily the clinical care of patients. It is essential from the beginning that these workers appreciate the importance of surveillance in the control of communicable diseases. The data collected must be simple and relevant. Constant feedback is necessary to maintain motivation.

One clinical worker in each health facility should be assigned the task of data collection and reporting, and if necessary be given on-site training. One person, normally assigned by the Ministry of Health, should be responsible for: (*a*) liaison with United Nations agencies and nongovernmental organizations, to collect data and report to the Ministry of Health, (*b*) analysing data from health facilities and (*c*) providing feedback. Each member of the surveillance team must have specified tasks to be completed within a defined time period.

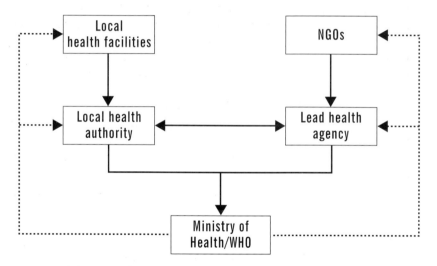

Figure 3.2   **Information flow for communicable disease surveillance in emergencies**

3.8.1   Health workers

This is the first contact that a sick person has with the health services. Reporting of data is only one of many tasks for the **clinical worker** at this level. Data must be simple and the number of items should be limited. Standard case definitions should be distributed and used for the diseases or syndromes under surveillance. Recording should be in line with clinical record-keeping practices. Tally sheets are very useful for this purpose. Suspected cases rather than confirmed cases should be reported. Zero reporting (when there are no cases) is also essential. Immediate reporting of an epidemic disease should be followed by an immediate response according to preset standard procedures.

In many emergency situations, there are **community workers** available for active case-finding, who can provide home treatment for mild cases and refer moderate or severe cases in a designated geographical area. These people, if trained, can increase the quality and completeness of the surveillance system.

Community key informants may be used to collect birth, death and migration information.

3.8.2   Health coordinator

At this level, data are collected from the health facilities (according to pre-arranged timing), usually under the responsibility of the health coordinator of the district/ area or agency. Distribution of forms and guidelines must be ensured by the health coordinator. The function of this level is the ongoing analysis of data in order to recognize outbreaks or changes in disease trends. Simple procedures should lead to an appropriate response such as investigation of suspected outbreaks. Organization for shipment and laboratory confirmation of samples from selected cases should be conducted at this level. Feedback of data to clinical workers is essential. Data should be reported to the Ministry of Health.

3.8.3   Ministry of health/head health agency

Data at this level should feed into the national surveillance system of the host country. The data can also be used for advocacy, fundraising, donor reports, programme reviews and overall evaluation of the effectiveness of health care interventions.

The tasks of the various health workers at key steps in surveillance are summarized in Table 3.9.

Table 3.9   **Tasks of health workers at key steps in surveillance**

Health worker	Detection	Reporting	Investigation		Analysis	Response		
			Laboratory	Epidemio-logy		Control	Policy	Feedback
Clinical worker	X	X	X			X		
Health coordinator		X	X	X	X	X	X	X
Ministry of Health/Lead health agency				X	X	X	X	X

3.9   Analysis and interpretation of surveillance data

Data analysis must be done at the field level by the health coordinator. In the initial stages of an emergency, the most important data elements to be analysed are the number of deaths and the number of victims of an emergency. Using these data, the crude mortality rate should be monitored daily during the acute phase. As those under 5 years of age are at higher risk of death in an emergency situation, mortality rate in this age group should also be calculated. If population data for the under-five age group are not available, an estimate of 17% of the total population may be used. For the under-fives, the cut-off value is more than 2/10 000 per day. The cut-off values for mortality in an emergency situation are shown in Table 3.10.

Table 3.10   **Crude mortality rate cut-off values in an emergency situation**

Phase	Crude mortality rate (deaths/10 000 population per day)	Under-five crude mortality rate (deaths/10 000 under-fives per day)
Normal	0.3–1.0	0.6–2.0
Alert	>1.0	> 2.0
Severe	> 2.0	> 4.0

For endemic diseases, morbidity trends over time are analysed by calculating incidence rates per 1000 population. For epidemic-prone diseases, particularly those for which one confirmed case constitutes an outbreak (e.g. cholera), absolute numbers of cases and attack rates must be analysed by place and person, i.e. location within the area and under 5, 5 and over, age groups. This information should be presented in a weekly report by the health coordinator in the emergency phase and then in a monthly report once the situation stabilizes. Simple summary tables, graphs and maps should be used as much as possible so that the information is readily understandable.

3.10 Feedback

3.10.1 Why feedback data?

Feedback is needed to:

* motivate clinical workers and give them an incentive to report data;
* inform health centre/clinical workers about the main health problems locally and at other health centres;
* provide examples of control measures: yellow fever vaccination, clean water, isolation, distribution of oral rehydration salts, new defecation field;
* feed forward to effect policy change.

One way to provide feedback of surveillance data is in a monthly epidemiological review (during an emergency, a weekly review is often required), which is a one-page summary of the major disease problems over the past month.

3.10.2 Performance indicators for the evaluation of a surveillance system

Reporting

Indicators of reporting are:

* zero reporting (see Section 3.6);
* timeliness:
  - percentage of weekly reports received within 48 hours of end of reporting period,
  - percentage of cases of epidemic prone diseases reported within 48 hours of onset of illness,
  - percentage of cases investigated within 48 hours of reporting of alert;
* completeness.

Laboratory efficiency

Indicators of laboratory efficiency may include, for example:

* the number of cholera cases for which samples were confirmed by the laboratory;
* the number of malaria cases confirmed by blood smear.

Investigation efficiency

Indicators of efficiency are periods/delays between:

* date of onset of the first case;
* date of reporting using outbreak alert form;
* date of investigation;
* date of response.

3.10.3 Further reading

Western KA. *Epidemiologic surveillance after natural disaster*. Washington, DC, Pan American Health Organization, 1982.

WHO recommended surveillance standards. Geneva, World Health Organization, 1999 (document WHO/EMC/DIS/97.1).

4. OUTBREAK CONTROL

This chapter outlines the key activities of outbreak control in an emergency on a step-by-step basis. An epidemic is the occurrence of a number of cases of a disease that is unusually large or unexpected for a given place and time. Outbreaks and epidemics refer to the same thing (although lay persons often regard outbreaks as small localized epidemics). The term outbreak will be used in this manual. Outbreaks can spread very rapidly in emergency situations and lead to high morbidity and mortality rates. The aim is to detect an outbreak as early as possible so as to control the spread of disease among the population at risk.

Control measures specific to different diseases are detailed under individual disease headings in Chapter 5.

It must never be forgotten that an increase in the number of cases of a disease may result from a sudden influx of displaced individuals. While this may not be an outbreak *stricto sensu* (that is to say, an increase in rate above a set value), it may nevertheless present the health services with a task equal to that of responding to an outbreak. Indeed, the task may be greater, since there may be a marked increase in the numbers of cases of several diseases rather than of a single disease and each of these may require a different response. This may not be an outbreak, but it may generate a medical emergency.

4.1 Preparedness

In each emergency situation, the lead agency for health is responsible for preparation for and response to a sharp increase in the numbers of cases of disease. To prepare for such an eventuality, it is essential that:

- a surveillance system is put in place to ensure early warning of an increase in the incidence or numbers of cases of diseases;
- an outbreak response plan is written for the disease – covering the resources, skills and activities required;
- standard treatment protocols for the disease are available to all health facilities and agencies and that clinical workers are trained;
- stockpiles of essential treatment supplies (medication and material) and laboratory sampling kits are available for the priority diseases, such as oral rehydration salts, intravenous fluids, vaccination material, tents, transport media and water purification supplies;
- a competent laboratory is identified for confirmation of cases;
- sources of relevant vaccines are identified in the event that a mass vaccination campaign is required, and that supplies of needles and syringes are adequate;

- sources of additional treatment supplies are identified for non vaccine-preventable diseases in case of expansion of outbreak;
- the availability and security of a cold chain are established.

There are a limited number of diseases with epidemic potential that pose a major threat to the health of a population facing an emergency situation (see Table 4.1). These diseases should be identified during the rapid assessment.

Table 4.1   **Major diseases with epidemic potential in emergency situations**

- Cholera
- Meningococcal disease
- Measles
- Shigellosis

In certain geographical areas, the following diseases may have to be included:
- Malaria
- Louse-borne typhus
- Yellow fever
- Trypanosomiasis
- Visceral or cutaneous leishmaniasis
- Viral haemorrhagic fevers
- Relapsing fever
- Typhoid
- Hepatitis A and E

In addition, the lead health agency should draw up a list of the main risk factors for outbreaks in the emergency-affected population. Potential risk factors are presented in Table 4.3.

A basic plan for resource requirements in the event of an outbreak should be developed (Table 4.4). For each disease, an outline response plan should be available on site.

Table 4.2   **SUMMARY: Steps in the management of a communicable disease outbreak**

---

1. PREPARATION
- Health coordination meetings.
- Surveillance system: weekly health reports to Ministry of Health and WHO (during an outbreak, this may be daily rather than weekly)
- Outbreak response plan for each disease: resources, skills and activities required.
- Stockpiles: sampling kits, appropriate antimicrobial, intravenous fluids, vaccines
- Contingency plans for isolation wards in hospitals (see Annex 7 for organization of an isolation centre).,
- Laboratory support.

2. DETECTION

The surveillance system must have an early warning mechanism for epidemic-prone diseases (see Annex 4 for guidelines on use of surveillance system and alert thresholds). If cases of any of the following diseases/syndromes are diagnosed (i.e. alert threshold is passed), inform the health coordinator as soon as possible; the health coordinator should inform the Ministry of Health and WHO:
- acute watery diarrhoea in over 5-year olds,
- bloody diarrhoea,
- suspected cholera,
- measles,
- meningitis,
- acute haemorrhagic fever syndrome,
- acute jaundice syndrome,
- suspected poliomyelitis (acute flaccid paralysis),
- a cluster of deaths of unknown origin,
(diseases/syndromes in list to be modified according to country profile).

Take clinical specimen (e.g. stool, serum, cerebrospinal fluid) for laboratory confirmation. Include case in weekly health report.

3. RESPONSE

Confirmation
- The lead health agency should investigate reported cases or alerts to confirm the outbreak situation – number of cases higher than expected for same period of year and population; clinical specimens will be sent for testing.
- The lead health agency should activate an outbreak control team with membership from relevant organizations: Ministry of Health, WHO and other United Nations organizations, nongovernmental organizations in the fields of health and water and sanitation, veterinary experts.

Investigation
- Confirm diagnosis (laboratory testing of samples).
- Define outbreak case definition.
- Count number of cases and determine size of population (to calculate attack rate).
- Collect/analyse descriptive data to date (e.g. time/date of onset, place/location of cases and individual characteristics such as age/sex).
- Determine the at-risk population.
- Formulate hypothesis for pathogen/source/transmission.
- Follow up cases and contacts.
- Conduct further investigation/epidemiological studies (e.g. to clarify mode of transmission, carrier, infectious dose required, better definition of risk factors for disease and at-risk groups.
- Write an investigation report (investigation results and recommendations for action).

Control
- Implement control and prevention measures specific for the disease.
- Prevent exposure (e.g. isolation of cases in cholera outbreak).
- Prevent infection (e.g. vaccination in measles outbreak).
- Treat cases with recommended treatment as in WHO/national guidelines.

4. EVALUATION

- Assess appropriateness and effectiveness of containment measures.
- Assess timeliness of outbreak detection and response..
- Change public health policy if indicated (e.g. preparedness).
- Write and disseminate outbreak report.

Table 4.3   Risk factors for outbreaks in emergency situations

Acute respiratory infections	Inadequate shelter with poor ventilation Indoor cooking, poor health care services Malnutrition, overcrowding Age group under 1 year old Large numbers of elderly Cold weather
Diarrhoeal diseases	Overcrowding Inadequate quantity and/or quality of water Poor personal hygiene Poor washing facilities Poor sanitation Insufficient soap Inadequate cooking facilities
Malaria	Movement of people from endemic into malaria-free zones or from areas of low endemicity to hyperendemic areas Interruption of vector control measures Increased population density promoting mosquito bites Stagnant water Inadequate health care services Flooding Changes in weather patterns
Measles	Measles vaccination coverage rates below 80% in country of origin, overcrowding, population displacement
Meningococcal meningitis	Meningitis belt (although the pattern is changing to include eastern, southern and central Africa) Dry season Dust storms Overcrowding High rates of acute respiratory infections
Tuberculosis	High HIV seroprevalence rates Overcrowding Malnutrition
Viral haemorrhagic fever	Contact with ape carcasses (filoviruses) Contact with wild-caught rodents (Lassa fever) Tick-infested areas (Crimea-Congo haemorrhagic fever) Poor infection control in health-care facilities
Louse-borne typhus	Highland areas Poor washing facilities Numerous body lice Endemic typhus/cases of Brill-Zinsser disease

---

Table 4.4   **Example of resources needed for outbreak response**

- Personnel (trained staff)
- Supplies (e.g. oral rehydration salts, intravenous fluids, water containers, water-purifying tablets, drinking cups, vaccines, vitamin A, monitoring forms, vaccination cards, tally sheets)
- Treatment facilities (location, beds available, stocks of basic medical supplies)
- Laboratory facilities (location, capacity, stocks of reagents, etc.)
- Transport (sources of emergency transport and fuel, cold chain)
- Communication links (between health centres; between Ministry of Health, nongovernmental organizations and United Nations agencies)
- Computers for data analysis
- In an outbreak requiring a vaccination campaign:
  - safe injection equipment (e.g. auto-destructible syringes and safety boxes (puncture-resistant boxes)
  - vaccination facilities (location, capacity)
  - cold chain equipment (number and condition of refrigerators, cold boxes, vaccine carriers, ice-packs)

4.2   Detection

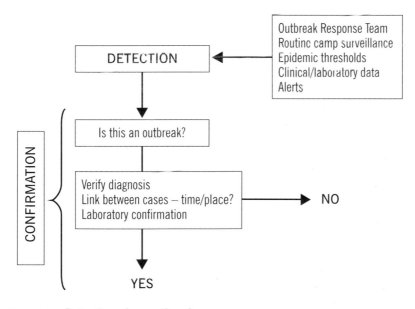

Figure 4.1   **Detection of an outbreak**

4.2.1   Surveillance

To ensure early detection of an outbreak in an emergency situation, a basic surveillance system with an early warning mechanism agreed by all operational agencies is essential. Reporting forms, case definitions and reporting mechanisms should be developed by the lead health agency at the beginning of the emergency and consensus reached with all agencies. Clinical workers at the primary and secondary care levels are the key component of this early warning system. They must be trained to report any suspected case of a disease with epidemic potential immediately to the health coordinator, using direct communication and/or the outbreak alert form (Annex 6).

To ensure rapid detection of an outbreak in an emergency situation, it will be necessary:

- to set up an early warning system within the surveillance system, with immediate reporting of diseases with epidemic potential;
- to train clinical workers to recognize priority diseases/syndromes;
- to train clinical workers to report cases of priority diseases/syndromes immediately to the health coordinator;
- for the health coordinator to report to the lead health agency;
- to arrange for enhanced surveillance during high-risk periods and in high-risk areas, e.g. for meningococcal meningitis during the dry season in the meningitis belt.

The analysis of these reports by the health coordinator will allow for the identification of clusters. It is vital that all suspected cases are followed up and verified. In camps established after large population displacements, an immediate response is necessary because of potentially high case attack rates and high mortality rates. Early detection can have a major impact in reducing the numbers of cases and deaths during an outbreak (see Fig. 4.2).

The surveillance system will ideally have detected an outbreak in the early stages. Once an outbreak occurs, investigation will be required to:

- confirm the outbreak,
- identify all cases and contacts,
- detect patterns of epidemic spread,
- estimate potential for further spread,
- determine whether control measures are working effectively.

Sequence of events in outbreak detection and confirmation: scenario 1

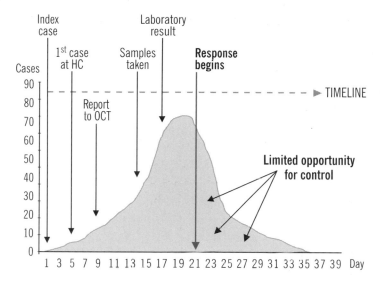

Sequence of events in outbreak detection and confirmation: scenario 2

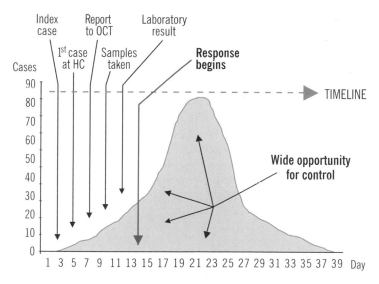

Figure 4.2   **The impact of early detection and response in reducing the disease burden caused by an outbreak in an emergency situation**

OCT: Outbreak control team

While routine surveillance depends on passive methods (i.e. the health workers report data weekly or monthly as part of their overall duties), in an outbreak there may be a need for active surveillance, where a member of the outbreak control team (OCT) specifically goes to the health facilities and reviews the records to detect further cases. This is particularly important for highly infectious diseases, such as viral haemorrhagic fever. Active case-finding may also be necessary where a home visitor goes into the community searching for further cases of the disease and refers to the health facility. Each case is then reported to the OCT.

The amount of data needed for each outbreak varies with the disease and the number of cases. In an explosive outbreak with large numbers of cases there will not be time to collect detailed information, so the priority is to collect numbers of cases and deaths on a line listing form. For outbreaks that are smaller in size or that evolve more slowly (such as a meningitis outbreak), a case investigation form should be completed for each case to obtain information such as contacts (see Annex 6).

4.2.2   Epidemic thresholds

The term epidemic threshold refers to the level of disease above which an urgent response is required. The threshold is specific to each disease and depends on the infectiousness, other determinants of transmission and local endemicity levels. For certain diseases, such as cholera or haemorrhagic fever, one case is sufficient to initiate a response. For other diseases, such as malaria, establishing a threshold ideally requires the collection of incidence data over a period of months or years.

However, most epidemic thresholds have been developed for stable populations, because these thresholds require longitudinal data over a period of years. There are few data on the use of these epidemic thresholds in emergency situations with recently displaced populations. Nevertheless, the establishment of a surveillance system early in an emergency situation will ensure that baseline data on diseases with epidemic potential are available. This will allow an assessment of whether an increase in numbers of cases or deaths requires action or not. At the onset of health activities, the health coordination team should set a threshold for each disease of epidemic potential above which an emergency response must be initiated (see Table 4.5).

Table 4.5   **Epidemic thresholds**

One suspected case of the following diseases represents a potential outbreak and requires immediate investigation:
- cholera
- measles
- typhus
- plague
- yellow fever
- viral haemorrhagic fever

An increase in the number of cases above a given threshold (or in numbers of cases per 1000 population) of the following diseases indicates a potential outbreak and requires immediate investigation:
- malaria
- shigellosis
- visceral leishmaniasis
- meningococcal meningitis
- human African trypanosomiasis
- others (e.g. typhoid fever, hepatitis A)

For areas of Africa where meningococcal disease is highly endemic, generic thresholds have been defined based on weekly surveillance of meningitis. Two thresholds are recommended to guide different sets of activities, depending on the phase of development of an outbreak.[2]

✔ The *alert threshold* is used to: (*a*) sound an early warning and launch an investigation at the start of an outbreak; (*b*) check epidemic preparedness; (*c*) start a vaccination campaign if there is an outbreak in a neighbouring area; and (*d*) prioritize areas for vaccination campaigns in the course of an outbreak. Sample alert thresholds are given in Annex 4.

✔ The *epidemic threshold* is used to confirm the emergence of an outbreak so as to step up control measures, i.e. mass vaccination and appropriate case management. The epidemic threshold depends on the context, and when the risk of an outbreak is high a lower threshold, more effective in this situation, is recommended (see Table 4.6).

Weekly meningitis incidence is calculated at health district level, for a population ranging from 30 000 to about 100 000 inhabitants. Incidence calculated for a large population (such as a city of more than 300 000 inhabitants) might not reach the threshold, even when the threshold is exceeded in some areas. In order to detect localized outbreaks, the region or city should be divided into areas of approximately 100 000 people for the purpose of calculating incidence.

For populations of less than 30 000, an absolute number of cases is used to define the alert and epidemic thresholds. This is to avoid major fluctuations in incidence owing to the small size of the population, and so as not to declare an outbreak too hastily on the basis of a small number of cases.

2 Detecting meningococcal meningitis epidemics in highly-endemic African countries: WHO recommendation. *Weekly Epidemiological Record*, 2000, 38:306–309.

Table 4.6   **Incidence thresholds for detection and control of epidemic meningococcal meningitis in highly endemic countries in Africa**

Intervention[a]	Population	
	> 30 000	**< 30 000**
Alert threshold • Inform authorities • Investigate • Confirm • Treat cases • Strengthen surveillance • Prepare	• Five cases per 100 000 inhabitants per week	• Two cases in 1 week *or* • An increase in the number of cases compared to previous non-epidemic years
Epidemic threshold • Mass vaccination • Distribute treatment to health centres • Treat according to epidemic protocol • Inform the public	If (1) no epidemic for 3 years and vaccination coverage < 80% or (2) alert threshold crossed early in the dry season: • 10 cases per 100 000 inhabitants per week In other situations: • 15 cases per 100 000 inhabitants per week	• Five cases in 1 week *or* • Doubling of the number of cases in a 3-week period *or* • Other situations should be studied on a case-by-case basis

[a] *If there is an epidemic in a neighbouring area, the alert threshold becomes the epidemic threshold.*

4.2.3   Outbreak control team (OCT)

Once the surveillance system detects an outbreak, or alerts have been received, the lead health agency must set up an OCT to investigate. Membership will essentially be similar to the health coordination team but may have to be expanded depending on the disease suspected and the control measures required. The OCT should include:

• a health coordinator,

• a clinical worker,

• a laboratory technician,

• a water/sanitation specialist,

• a vector control specialist,

• a representative of the local health authority,

• health educators,

• community leaders.

One member of the team should be the team leader; this is usually the health coordinator of the lead health agency. Each agency should be given a clear role for response to an outbreak, such as the establishment of an isolation centre or the implementation of a mass vaccination programme.

In the event of a suspected outbreak, the OCT must:

- meet daily to review the latest data on suspected cases/deaths and follow up any alerts;
- implement the outbreak response plan (see preparedness section) for the disease covering the resources, skills and activities required;
- identify sources of additional human and material resources for managing the outbreak, e.g. treatment sites in a cholera outbreak;
- define the tasks of each member in managing the outbreak, e.g. surveillance, vaccination;
- ensure the use of standard treatment protocols for the disease by all agencies and train clinical workers if necessary;
- coordinate with the local heath authorities, nongovernmental organizations and United Nations agencies.

4.3 Confirmation

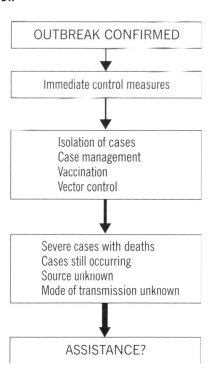

Figure 4.3   **Confirmation of an outbreak**

4.3.1 Verification of an outbreak and laboratory confirmation

Reports and alerts of outbreaks are frequent in emergency situations and must always be followed up. It is important to aware that in some languages one word may be used for more than one disease (e.g. in Serbo-Croat and its variants the same word is used for typhus and typhoid). Diagnosis must be confirmed either on a clinical basis by senior clinical workers (e.g. for measles) or by laboratory tests, in which case specimens (e.g. blood, serum, faeces or cerebrospinal fluid) must be sent to a laboratory for testing. Material required for an outbreak investigation is listed in Annex 6.

An assessment of current clinical and epidemiological information is the starting point for dealing with the problem of an outbreak of unknown origin. The historical knowledge of regional endemic and epidemic diseases, as well as their seasonality, further defines the possible causes. Since a variety of infectious agents can cause a similar clinical picture, the initial steps of the outbreak investigation (case definitions, questionnaires, etc.) should generally elaborate on known syndromes (e.g. fever of unknown origin, acute neurological syndrome, acute jaundice) rather than on any preconceived diagnosis. One or more specimen types may be required to define the cause of the outbreak.

Laboratory confirmation of initial cases is necessary for most diseases when an outbreak is suspected. There must be an efficient mechanism for getting the correct samples in good condition from the patient to the laboratory and getting the result back to the OCT and clinical workers. At the onset of health care activities in a camp, the lead health agency must set out the method for sampling, the type of samples to be taken and the tests to be undertaken, and identify the relevant laboratories with complete addresses. The agency must assess the diagnostic capability of the local laboratory, including the availability of rapid diagnostic kits. A reference laboratory must also be identified at regional or international level to test, for example, for the antimicrobial sensitivity of *Shigella* spp. Table 4.7 outlines the steps in laboratory confirmation.

Table 4.7 **Steps in laboratory confirmation**

Collection of samples	Sampling equipment, specimen containers, training of clinical workers in sampling techniques
Transport of samples	On-site/referral laboratory
Safe packaging	Appropriate leak-proof transport containers
Testing samples	Quality assurance in laboratory
Reporting result	When, to whom
Interpreting result	Implications for control measures

If a certain pathogen, source or mode of transmission is suspected, **control measures should not be delayed** if laboratory confirmation is not yet available. In the absence of laboratory confirmation, epidemiological information should continue to be collected, as this will facilitate the initial control measures.

Table 4.8   **Laboratory specimens required for tests for specific causative agents**

Suspected disease	Specimen	Diagnostic test	Additional information needed
Cholera	Fresh stool/ rectal swab in transport medium	Culture	Antimicrobial sensitivity testing
Hepatitis B	Serum (+4 °C)	Antigen detection	
Malaria	Blood (thick and thin smears)	Staining Rapid diagnostic tests (for *P. falciparum* and *P. vivax*)	
Meningococcal meningitis	CSF[a] Blood	Gram stain Rapid diagnostic test	Serogrouping
Shigellosis	Fresh stool/ rectal swab in transport medium	Culture Rapid diagnostic test	Serogrouping Antimicrobial sensitivity testing
Typhoid fever	Blood in culture bottles	Culture	
Typhus	Serum (+4 °C)	Serology	
Viral haemorrhagic fevers	Blood	Antigen detection	

Note: Measles is diagnosed clinically and does not require laboratory confirmation.
[a] CSF: cerebrospinal fluid

4.3.2   Planning for specimen collection

After the clinical syndrome and suspect pathogen(s) have been defined, the clinical specimens for collection and appropriate laboratory diagnosis should be determined (Table 4.8).

In the event of an outbreak, one agency should coordinate the transport of specimens and follow up on the results of laboratory tests. Laboratories with the capacity to test (a) stool samples for *Shigella*, *Salmonella* and cholera and (b) CSF samples for meningococci should be identified rapidly. WHO maintains an updated database of international reference laboratories for testing of stool samples for poliovirus, or serum samples for dengue fever, Japanese encephalitis and agents of viral haemorrhagic fevers.

4.3.3   Specimen collection and processing

Specimens obtained in the acute phase of the disease, preferably before administration of antimicrobial drugs, are more likely to yield laboratory identification of the cause. Before specimen collection begins, the procedure should be explained to the patient and his/her relatives. The appropriate precautions for safety during collection and processing of samples must be followed.

Procedures for collection of specific specimens are detailed in Annex 8.

Labelling and identification of specimens

In an outbreak investigation, the information contained in the case investigation and laboratory request forms is collected along with the specimen. Each patient should be assigned a unique identification number by the collection team. It is the link between the laboratory results on the line listing form, the specimens and the patient, which guides further investigation and response to the outbreak. This unique identification number should be present and used as a common reference together with the patient's name on all specimens, epidemiological databases, and forms for case investigation or laboratory request.

Label specimen container/slide

Labels (at least five) should be used whenever possible. The label should be permanently affixed to the specimen container. It should contain:

• the patient's name,
• the unique identification number,
• the specimen type and date and place of collection,
• the name or initials of the specimen collector.

Case investigation and laboratory forms

A case investigation form should be completed for each patient at the time of collection. The originals remain with the investigation team, and should be kept together for analysis and later reference. A laboratory form must also be completed for each specimen. The epidemiological and clinical data gathered in the investigation can then easily be tied to the laboratory results for analysis later.

The form includes:

• patient information: age (or date of birth), sex, complete address,
• clinical information: date of onset of symptoms, clinical and vaccination history, risk factors, antimicrobials taken before collection of specimens,
• laboratory information: acute or convalescent specimen, other specimens from the same patient.

The form must also record the date and time when the specimen was taken and when it was received by the laboratory, and the name of the person collecting the specimen.

4.3.4   Storage of specimens

To preserve bacterial or viral viability in specimens for microbiological culture or inoculation, specimens should be placed in appropriate media and stored at recommended temperatures. These conditions must be preserved throughout transport to the laboratory and will vary according to transportation time. They will differ for different specimens and pathogens, depending on their sensitivity to desiccation, temperature, nutrient and pH.

Many specimens taken for viral isolation are viable for 2 days if maintained in type-specific media at 4–8 °C. These specimens must be frozen only as directed by expert advice, as infectivity may be altered.

Specimens for bacterial culture should be kept in appropriate transport media at the recommended temperature. This ensures bacterial viability while minimizing overgrowth of other microorganisms. With the exception of cerebrospinal fluid, urine and sputum, most specimens may be kept at ambient temperature if they will be processed within 24 hours. For periods > 24 hours, storage at 4–8 °C is advisable except for particularly cold-sensitive organisms such as *Shigella* spp., meningococcus and pneumococcus. These exceptions must be kept at ambient temperature. Longer delays are not advisable, as the yield of bacteria may fall significantly.

Specimens for antigen or antibody detection may be stored at 4–8 °C for 24–48 hours, or at –20 °C for longer periods. Sera for antibody detection may be stored at 4–8 °C for up to 10 days. Although not ideal, room temperature may still be useful for storing serum samples for antibody testing, even for prolonged periods (weeks). Thus samples that have been collected should not be discarded simply because there are no refrigeration facilities available.

Transport of specimens requires appropriate safety boxes, cold boxes and coolant blocks and may require a suitable cold chain.

4.4   Response

4.4.1   Investigation of source and modes of transmission

The OCT should:

* meet daily to update the team on outbreak developments;
* review the human, logistic (stores, stocks, etc.) and financial resources available to manage the outbreak;
* oversee the investigation of reported cases to assess pathogen, source and transmission;
* ensure that clinical workers report suspected cases to the team immediately;
* ensure that clinical workers are using standard treatment protocols;

- ensure that cases are quantified by time and place;
- produce spot maps and epidemic curves;
- oversee the implementation of control measures.

Collection and analysis of descriptive data and development of hypotheses

The systematic recording of data on cases and deaths (time, place and person) in an outbreak is essential to ensure accurate reporting. These data are necessary to form a hypothesis of the pathogen involved and its source and route of transmission, and to measure the effectiveness of control measures. This process is summarized in the six key questions: Who? What? When? Where? Why? How?

A simple, clear, easily understood case definition must be used consistently from the beginning of an outbreak and must be placed conspicuously at the top of each case reporting form. This case definition, the *outbreak case definition*, may have to be adapted from the surveillance case definition. The syndromic definitions often used by the surveillance system for early detection may not be sufficiently specific in the event of an outbreak and could lead to an overestimation of cases. In most outbreaks, basic epidemiological data on time, place, person and basic laboratory confirmation are sufficient for the design and implementation of effective control measures.

Cases may be placed in two categories: suspected or confirmed. A suspected case is one in which the clinical signs and symptoms are compatible with the disease in question but laboratory confirmation of infection is lacking (negative or pending). A confirmed case is one in which there is definite laboratory evidence of current or recent infection, *whether or not* clinical signs or symptoms are or have been present. Once laboratory investigations have confirmed the diagnosis in the initial cases, the use of a clinical/epidemiological case definition may be sufficient and there may be no need to continue to collect laboratory specimens from new cases for the purposes of notification.

During an epidemic, data should be analysed rapidly to determine the extent of the outbreak and the impact of actions taken to date (Fig. 4.4).

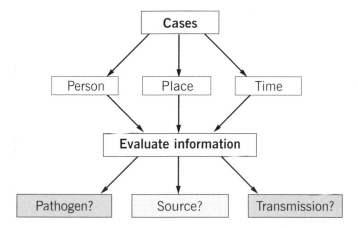

Figure 4.4   **Collection and analysis of descriptive data**

The following steps should be taken by members of the outbreak control team in charge of the epidemiological investigation.

- Define the extent of the outbreak in time, place and person:
  - when did the cases occur – dates of onset (e.g. epidemic curve)?
  - where do cases live (e.g. spot map)?
  - who are they (e.g. tables of age, vaccination status)?
- Measure the severity of the outbreak:
  - how many cases were hospitalized?
  - how many cases suffered complications?
  - how many cases died as a proportion of all cases (case-fatality rate)?
- Draw an epidemic curve, i.e. a graph showing cases by date of onset. This helps to demonstrate where and how an outbreak began, how quickly the disease is spreading, the stage of the outbreak (start, middle or end phase) and whether control efforts are having an impact (Fig. 4.4).
- Draw a graph or table of age distribution and vaccination status of cases; this should be constructed from the line listing of cases. This information is used for identifying cases that were not preventable (e.g. those developing measles before the scheduled age of vaccination). If population data are available, calculate age-specific attack rates.
- If appropriate, estimate the vaccine efficacy. In the case of a vaccine-preventable disease such as measles, vaccine efficacy and the proportion of cases that were vaccine-preventable should be calculated. Using vaccination history data it is possible to tabulate those immunized but not protected (vaccine failures) and those who failed to be immunized.

- Draw a spot map. A map of the camp or community should be marked with the location of all cases and deaths. The outbreak control team can use this map to identify areas with clusters of disease. Further investigation of these areas may reveal the source of infection or modes of transmission. Even when a camp is involved, it is essential that the effect on the local community outside the camp is documented (this may be the source) and the local health authorities assisted in controlling the outbreak if it has spread.

- Provide summary data of the outbreak, by calculating the basic epidemiological indices set out in Table 4.9.

Table 4.9   **Basic epidemiological indices**

The case-fatality rate (CFR) is the percentage of cases that result in death
- Count the number of cases who died of the disease
- Divide by the total number of cases of the disease
- Multiply the result by 100

The weekly attack rate is the number of cases per 10 000 people per week
- Divide 10 000 by the total emergency-affected population
- Multiply the result by the number of cases that occurred in a given week

---

The age-specific weekly attack rate is the number of cases per 10 000 people in one age group (e.g. > 5 years)
- Calculate the number of persons in that age group in the camp
- Count the number of cases in the age group for the chosen week
- Divide 10 000 by the number of persons
- Multiply the result by the number of cases in that group

Follow-up of cases and contacts

For each case, information should be collected on name, age, location, date of onset and outcome; for some diseases, additional information on vaccination status, water source and duration of disease may be collected.

An alert registry must be established to record alerts of cases systematically. One site should be dedicated to this activity. The registry must have close links to home visitors and the local community and its existence must be widely advertised. It should be carefully maintained and used to provide material for the team.

Active case-finding may be required, depending on the infectiousness of the disease and the risk to the population. Contact-tracing may also be required, particularly in the case of outbreaks of viral haemorrhagic fever. The OCT must define what constitutes a contact, specify the period of risk and agree on the method of follow-up, e.g. active contact-tracing.

Further investigation/epidemiological studies

In some outbreaks, routine data do not give sufficient information about items such as the source of the outbreak, risk factors, local characteristics of the causative agent (e.g. resistance, serotype) or mode of transmission. Further investigation, such as case control studies or environmental assessments (e.g. vector breeding sites), may be required to identify the source of this outbreak, risk factors in respect of severity, or modes of transmission. This may need the participation of external agencies with skills in epidemiological investigation or in specific diseases.

4.4.2   Control

The data gathered in the course of these investigations should reveal why the outbreak occurred and the mechanisms by which it spread. These in turn, together with what is known about the epidemiology and biology of the organism involved, will make it possible to define the measures needed to control the outbreak and prevent further problems.

An outbreak may be controlled by eliminating or reducing the source of infection, interrupting transmission and protecting persons at risk. In the initial stage of an outbreak in an emergency situation, the exact nature of the causative agent may not be known and general control measures may have to be taken for a suspected cause. Once the cause is confirmed, specific measures such as vaccination can be undertaken. These disease-specific measures are detailed in Chapter 5.

Control strategies fall into four major categories of activity.

1. *Prevention of exposure*: the source of infection is reduced to prevent the disease spreading to other members of the community. Depending on the disease, this may involve prompt diagnosis and treatment of cases using standard protocols (e.g. cholera), isolation and barrier nursing of cases (e.g. viral haemorrhagic fevers), health education, improvements in environmental and personal hygiene (e.g. cholera, typhoid fever, shigellosis, hepatitis A and hepatitis E), control of the animal vector or reservoir (e.g. malaria, dengue, yellow fever, Lassa fever) and proper disposal of sharp instruments (e.g., hepatitis B).

2. *Prevention of infection*: susceptible groups are protected by vaccination (e.g. meningitis, yellow fever and measles), safe water, adequate shelter and good sanitation.

3. *Prevention of disease*: high-risk groups are offered chemoprophylaxis (e.g. malaria prophylaxis may be suggested for pregnant women in outbreaks) and better nutrition.

4. *Prevention of death*: through prompt diagnosis and management of cases, effective health care services (e.g. acute respiratory infections, malaria, bacterial dysentery, cholera, measles, meningitis).

Selection of control measures depends on:
- feasibility (technical/operational),
- availability (stockpiles),
- acceptability,
- safety (of operators and population),
- cost.

Patient isolation

The degree of isolation required depends on the infectiousness of the disease. Strict barrier isolation is rarely indicated in health facilities, except for outbreaks of highly infectious diseases such as viral haemorrhagic fevers. The isolation room must be in a building separate from other patient areas and access must be strictly limited. Good ventilation with screened doors is ideal, but fans should be avoided as they raise dust and droplets and can spread aerosols. Biohazard warning notices must be placed at the entrances to patients' rooms. Patients must remain isolated until they have fully recovered.

During outbreaks, isolation of patients or of those suspected of having the disease can reinforce stigmatization and hostile behaviour of the public toward ill persons. The establishment of isolation rules in a community or in a health facility is not a decision to be taken lightly, and should always be accompanied by careful information and education of all members of the involved community. Every isolated patient should be allowed to be attended by at least one family member. Provided that enough supplies are available, designated family attendants should receive barrier nursing equipment, and be instructed on how to protect themselves when in contact with the patient.

Every outbreak requires a response specific to the disease. Control measures for the main communicable diseases encountered by displaced populations are described under disease-specific sections in Chapter 5.

Biohazardous materials

Safe disposal of body fluids and excreta is essential, especially in the case of highly contagious diseases. This may be achieved by disinfecting with bleach or by incineration. If contaminated material has to be transported, it should be placed in a double bag.

The threat of infection from body fluids of patients with diseases such as cholera, shigellosis or viral haemorrhagic fevers is serious, and strict procedures for disposal of hazardous waste must be maintained. Laboratory specimens and contaminated equipment should also be carefully sterilized or disposed of. When possible, heating methods such as autoclaving, incineration or boiling can be used to disinfect. Proper disposal of sharp objects such as needles is essential.

Table 3.10 outlines the general precautions to be taken in relation to isolation of cases. See Section 2.3.6 for procedures for the disposal of the dead.

Table 3.10   **General precautions to be taken for isolation of cases in outbreaks**

Isolation measure	Contagious-ness of cases	Route of transmission	Type of protective measure	Diseases
Standard precautions	Moderate	Direct or indirect contact with faeces, urine, blood, body fluids and contaminated articles	Hand-washing, safe disposal of contaminated articles	Most infectious diseases except those mentioned below
Enteric isolation	High	Direct contact with patients and with faeces and oral secretions	Contact precautions	Cholera, shigellosis, typhoid fever Gastroenteritis caused by rotavirus, *E. coli,* hepatitis A
Respiratory isolation	High	Direct contact with patients or oral secretions and droplets	Separate room, masks, contact precautions	Meningococcal meningitis, diphtheria, measles
Strict isolation	Very high	Airborne Direct contact with infected bloods, secretions, organs or semen	Separate room, biohazard notification	Viral haemorrhagic fevers

Prompt diagnosis and effective case management

There are two steps in this process: timely presentation to the health facility and effective diagnosis and treatment by the clinical workers. Home visitors and health educators can play an important role in ensuring that the community is aware of the symptoms and signs a disease, and that they know that effective treatment is available at the health facility. The second step is the use of standard treatment protocols by clinical workers well trained in their use. The early diagnosis of a disease is important, not only to avoid serious sequelae and death in the patient but also to prevent further transmission.

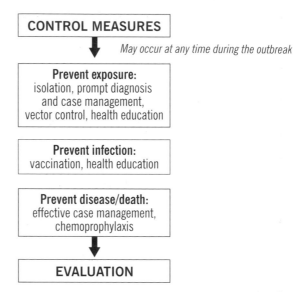

Figure 4.5   **Control strategies for an outbreak**

4.5   Evaluation

After an outbreak, the outbreak control team must carry out a thorough evaluation of the following:

- cause of the outbreak,
- surveillance and detection of the outbreak,
- preparedness for the outbreak,
- management of the outbreak,
- control measures.

The specific issues under each heading that should be evaluated include:

- timeliness of detection and response,
- effectiveness,
- cost,
- lost opportunities,
- new/revised policies.

The findings of this evaluation should be documented in a written report containing clear recommendations on:

- the epidemiological characteristics of the epidemic,
- surveillance,
- preparedness,
- control measures carried out.

Evaluation should feed back into preparedness activities for future outbreaks.

4.5.1. Further reading

Basic laboratory methods in medical parasitology. Geneva, World Health Organization, 1991.

Bench aids for the diagnosis of malaria infections. Geneva, World Health Organization, 2000.

Cheesbrough M. *District laboratory practice in tropical countries, Part 1*. Cambridge, Cambridge University Press, 1998.

Cheesbrough M. *District laboratory practice in tropical countries, Part 2*. Cambridge, Cambridge University Press, 2000.

El-Nageh MM. *Specimen collection and transport for microbiological investigation*. Alexandria, WHO Regional Office for the Eastern Mediterranean, 1994 (WHO Regional Publications, Eastern Mediterranean Series, No. 8).

El-Nageh MM et al. *Health laboratory facilities in emergency and disaster situations*. Alexandria, WHO Regional Office for the Eastern Mediterranean, 1994 (WHO Regional Publications, Eastern Mediterranean Series, No. 5).

Guidelines for the safe transport of infectious substances and diagnostic specimens. Geneva, World Health Organization, 1997 (document WHO/EMC/97.3).

Guidelines for the collection of clinical specimens during field investigation of outbreaks. Geneva, World Health Organization, 2000 (document WHO/CDS/CSR/EDC/2000.4).

Infection control for viral haemorrhagic fevers in the African health care setting. Geneva, World Health Organization, 1998 (document WHO/EMC/ESR/98.2).

Johns W, El-Nageh MM. *Selection of basic laboratory equipment for laboratories with limited resources*. Geneva, World Health Organization, 2000.

Reingold AL. Outbreak investigations – a perspective. *Emerging Infectious Diseases*, 1998, **4**(1):21–27.

5. DISEASE PREVENTION AND CONTROL

5.1 Acute respiratory infections

Basic facts

- Acute respiratory infections can involve:
    - the upper respiratory tract – common cold, otitis media and pharyngitis;
    - the lower respiratory tract – bronchitis, bronchiolitis and pneumonia.
- The majority of acute respiratory infections involve the upper respiratory tract only, are mild and resolve spontaneously.
- Acute lower respiratory tract infections (LRTIs) are a major cause of mortality and morbidity in emergency situations.
- Some 25%–30% of deaths in children under 5 years of age are due to LRTIs; 90% of these deaths are due to pneumonia.
- It is therefore important that pneumonia is recognized quickly and treated appropriately. A simplified approach adapted to primary health care is indicated in Annex 11.
- Causative organisms may be bacterial (mainly *Haemophilus influenzae* and *Streptococcus pneumoniae*) or viral.
- Risk factors for pneumonia include low birth weight, malnutrition, vitamin A deficiency, poor breastfeeding practices, bad ventilation in shelters, chilling in infants and overcrowding.

Case management

- Priority should be given to early recognition and adequate treatment of pneumonia.
- All children presenting with cough and/or difficult breathing should be carefully assessed.
- Signs of malnutrition should also be assessed, as this increases the risk of death from pneumonia.
- Severely malnourished children must be referred to hospital.
- Management of pneumonia consists of antimicrobial therapy.
- Choice of antimicrobial depends on national protocols and available drugs.
- The New Emergency Health Kits (see Annex 10) contain co-trimoxazole, which covers a broad spectrum of bacterial agents of pneumonia and is cost-effective.
- Alternatives are amoxicillin and chloramphenicol.

- For severe pneumonia, injectable antimicrobial such as penicillin, ampicillin or chloramphenicol should be used.
- Supportive measures, such as oral fluids to prevent dehydration, continued feeding to avoid malnutrition, antipyretics to reduce fever and protection from cold, are essential.
- Vaccination against measles, diphtheria and whooping cough is effective in reducing the impact of acute respiratory infections.
- Table 3 of Annex 11 lists treatment guidelines using the most commonly available antimicrobial: co-trimoxazole, amoxicillin and procaine penicillin.

Further reading

Acute respiratory infections in children: case management in small hospitals in developing countries. A manual for doctors and other senior health workers. Geneva, World Health Organization, 1992 (document WHO/ARI/90.5).

WHO-UNICEF joint statement on Management of pneumonia in community settings. World Health Organization, 2004 (WHO/FCH/CAH/04.06).

5.2 Bacillary dysentery (shigellosis)

Basic facts

- Bacillary dysentery is an acute bacterial disease involving the large and small intestine.
- It is caused by bacteria of the genus *Shigella*, of which *S. dysenteriae* type 1 causes the most severe disease and the largest outbreaks (other species include *S. flexneri, S. sonnei* and *S. boydii*).
- It is the most important cause of acute bloody diarrhoea.

Shigella dysenteriae **type 1**

- The disease is most severe in young children, the elderly and the malnourished.
- Displaced populations are at high risk in situations of overcrowding, poor sanitation and limited access to safe water.
- In an outbreak, up to one-third of the population at risk may be infected.
- Transmission occurs through contaminated food and water and from person to person.
- The disease is highly contagious – the infective dose is only 10–100 organisms.
- Treatment is with antimicrobials, which decrease the severity and reduce the duration of illness.
- The disease is not usually associated with a marked loss of fluid and electrolytes.
- Without prompt, effective treatment the case-fatality rate can be as high as 10%.

Apart from *S. dysenteriae* type 1 and other *Shigella* species, dysentery can be caused by *Campylobacter jejuni*, entero-invasive *Escherichia coli*, *Salmonella* and, less frequently, *Entamoeba histolytica*.

Types of patients at high risk of contracting bacillary dysentery are listed in Table 5.1.

Table 5.1 **High-risk patients**

• Children under 5 years of age, and especially infants, severely malnourished children and children who have had measles in the past 6 weeks
• Older children and adults who are obviously malnourished
• Patients who are severely dehydrated, have had a convulsion, or are seriously ill when first seen
• Adults 50 years of age or older

Clinical features

- Bloody diarrhoea is often associated with fever, abdominal cramps and rectal pain.
- The incubation period is usually 1–3 days, but may be up to 1 week for *S. dysenteriae* type 1 infection.
- Complications include sepsis, rectal prolapse, haemolytic uraemic syndrome and seizures.

Diagnosis

- Blood is observed in a fresh stool specimen.
- *S. dysenteriae* type 1 is isolated from stool samples (see Annex 8 for stool sampling and transport procedures).

Case management

- Refer seriously ill or severely malnourished patients to hospital immediately.
- Check the results of antimicrobial sensitivity tests with the laboratory.
- Give an antimicrobial effective against local *S. dysenteriae* type 1 (Sd1) strains promptly to all patients, preferably as inpatients (see Table 5.2).
- Treat dehydration with oral rehydration salts or intravenous fluids if severe.
- If the antimicrobials used are effective, clinical improvement should be noted within 48 hours.
- If antimicrobials used are effective, clinical improvement should be noted within 48 hours. Treatment with ciprofloxacin should be given for 3 days.

IMPORTANT. Do not give antimicrobials known to be ineffective. The antimicrobial used should be in line with national guidelines and selected on the basis of susceptibility testing of local Sd1 strains.

When the supply of an effective antimicrobial is limited, priority should be given to high-risk patients (see Table 5.1).

Table 5.2   **Recommended antibiotics for treatment of *Shigella dysenteriae* type 1**

ADULTS: ciprofloxacin	500 mg	twice a day	by mouth for 3 days
CHILDREN: ciprofloxacin	15 mg/kg	twice a day	by mouth for 3 days
FOR CHILDREN AGED UNDER 6 MONTHS: add zinc	zinc 10 mg	daily	by mouth for 2 weeks
FOR CHILDREN AGED 6 MONTHS TO 3 YEARS: add zinc	zinc 20 mg	daily	by mouth for 2 weeks

Note: rapidly evolving antimicrobial resistance is a real problem. Shigella is usually resistant to ampicillin and trimethoprim sulfamethoxazole (TMP-SMX)

Further reading

Guidelines for the control of shigellosis including epidemics due to Shigella dysenteriae *type 1.* World Health Organization 2005 (ISBN 92 4 159533 0).

The management of bloody diarrhoea in young children. Geneva, World Health Organization, 1994 (document WHO/CDR/94.49).

5.3   Cholera

Basic facts

- Cholera is an acute bacterial enteric disease caused by the Gram-negative bacillus *Vibrio cholerae.*
- *Vibrio cholerae* produces a powerful enterotoxin that causes profuse watery diarrhoea by a secretory mechanism.
- Infection results from ingestion of organisms in food and water, or directly from person to person by the faecal–oral route.

- Acute carriers, including those with asymptomatic or mild disease, are important in the maintenance and transmission of cholera.

- It is asymptomatic in more than 90% of cases.

- Attack rates in displaced populations can be as high as 10–15% (e.g. Goma, Democratic Republic of Congo in 1994), whereas in normal situations it is estimated at 1–2%.

- Case-fatality rates are usually around 5% but have reached 40% in large outbreaks in refugee camps (e.g. Goma, Democratic Republic of Congo in 1994).

- With appropriate treatment (oral rehydration in most cases) the case-fatality rate can be reduced to 1% or less.

Clinical features

- The incubation period is usually between 1 and 5 days.

- Symptoms begin with the abrupt onset of copious watery diarrhoea, classically rice-water stools, with or without vomiting.

- Loss of water and electrolytes can lead to rapid and profound dehydration, low serum potassium levels and acidosis.

- Fever is unusual, except in children.

- Vomiting without associated nausea may develop, usually after the onset of diarrhoea.

- Severe dehydration leads to loss of skin turgor, malaise, tachypnoea and hypotension.

Early detection of cholera is important to ensure prompt treatment and reduction of environmental contamination. Cholera should be suspected when:

- a patient over 5 years of age develops severe dehydration from acute watery diarrhoea (usually with vomiting); or

- any patient over 2 years of age has acute watery diarrhoea *in an area where there is an outbreak of cholera.*

Diagnosis

- Isolation of *Vibrio cholerae* O1 or O139 from stools is still the only acceptable standard for confirmation of cholera.

- Rapid point-of-care diagnostic tests on stool samples are available in some countries, but no data exist on their performance under field condition. Their use might be considered in the future, as validation and standardization become better documented.

(See Annex 8 for stool sampling and transport procedures.)

Case management

- The prevention and treatment of dehydration are the mainstay of cholera management (Annex 12).

- The use of antimicrobials (doxycycline/tetracycline) is not essential for the treatment of cholera but may be recommended to reduce the volume of diarrhoea and shorten the duration of excretion. In emergencies, systematic administration of antimicrobials is justified only for severe cases and in situations where bed occupancy, patient turnover or stocks of intravenous fluids are expected to reach critical levels in respect of case management capacity.
- Treatment is single dose of doxycycline 300 mg or tetracycline for 3 days.
- A sensitivity profile of the outbreak strain must be available as soon as possible to decide on the possible choice of antimicrobial for severe cases. Oral antimicrobials only must be given, and after the patient has been rehydrated (usually in 4–6 hours) and vomiting has stopped.

Prevention and control measures

- Prompt diagnosis and appropriate treatment of patients must be carried out.
- Cholera treatment centres should be established, with barrier nursing procedures specific to enteric pathogens (see Annex 7 for organization of an isolation centre, essential rules in a CTC, disinfectant preparation, and calculation of treatment needs).
- Faecal material and vomit must be properly disinfected and disposed of.
- Health education programmes should be conducted on hygiene and disinfection measures with simple messages on safe water, safe food and hand-washing.
- Funerals should be held quickly and near the place of death.
- Those who prepare the body for burial must be meticulous about washing their hands with soap and clean water.
- Promote washing of hands with soap and clean water whenever food is being handled.

Inappropriate control measures

- Mass chemoprophylaxis has never succeeded in limiting the spread of cholera.
- Trade and travel restrictions do not prevent the spread of cholera and are unnecessary. (See Section 2.6.7 for use of new oral cholera vaccines.)

Further reading

Sanchez JL, Taylor DN. Cholera. *Lancet*, 1997, **349**(9068):1825–1830.

Cholera outbreak: assessing the outbreak response and improving preparedness. World Health Organization, 2004. (document WHO/CDS/CPE/ZFK/2004.4)

First steps for managing an outbreak of acute diarrhoea. World Health Organization, 2004 (document WHO/CDS/NCS/2003.7 Rev 1).

Acute diarrhoeal diseases in complex emergencies: critical steps. World Health Organization, 2004 (document WHO/CDS/CPE/ZFK/2004.6).

5.4   Other diarrhoeal diseases

Basic facts

Diarrhoeal diseases are a major cause of morbidity and mortality in emergency situations, mainly because of inadequate water supply in terms of quality and quantity, insufficient, poorly maintained sanitation facilities and overcrowding. In camp situations, diarrhoeal diseases have accounted for more than 40% of deaths in the acute phase of the emergency. Over 80% of deaths are among children under 2 years of age.

Common sources of infection are shown in Table 5.3.

Table 5.3   **Common sources of infection in emergency situations**

Outbreak investigations in emergency situations have identified the following risk factors for infection:
- polluted water sources (e.g. by faecally contaminated surface water entering an incompletely sealed well), or contamination during storage or transport (e.g. by contact with hands soiled by faeces);
- shared water containers and cooking pots;
- lack of soap;
- contaminated food items (e.g. dried fish, shellfish).

Clinical features

Diarrhoea is defined as three or more abnormally loose or fluid stools over a period of 24 hours. Bacteria such as *Salmonella* (commonly *S*. Enteritidis or *S*. Typhimurium) and *Escherichia coli* can cause diarrhoea, but the most severe outbreaks are caused by *Shigella dysenteriae* type 1 and *Vibrio cholerae* (see Sections 5.2 and 5.3). Other pathogens that cause diarrhoea include protozoa (such as *Giardia lamblia, E. histolytica, C. parvum*) and viruses (such as rotavirus and Norwalk virus). Diarrhoea may occur as one of the symptoms of other infections (e.g. measles).

The major complications of diarrhoea are dehydration and the negative effect on nutritional status.

Diagnosis

The diagnosis of diarrhoeal diseases is usually based on clinical signs and symptoms. However, in outbreak situations stool samples must be collected from 10–20 cases to confirm the cause and to identify antimicrobial sensitivity. Once the outbreak has been confirmed, it is not necessary to obtain laboratory confirmation for every patient as this depletes laboratory supplies.

IMPORTANT. Do not wait for laboratory results before starting treatment/control activities.

Case management

For assessment and case management of diarrhoea, see Annex 12.

Prevention and control measures

The prevention of diarrhoeal diseases depends on the provision and use of safe water, adequate sanitation and health education (see Table 5.4). An adequate water supply is essential to protect health and is one of the highest priorities for camp planners. A supply of adequate quantities of water (reasonably clean if possible) in emergency situations is more important than a supply of small quantities of microbiologically pure water.

Table 5.4   **Key components in the prevention of diarrhoeal diseases**

Practices or activities	Interventions to move theory to practice
Safe drinking-water	Provision of an adequate supply, collection, transport and storage system
	Provision of information on the importance of clean water with appropriate use of water container lids and household storage
Safe disposal of human excreta	Provision of adequate facilities for the disposal of human waste
	Provision of information on the importance of human waste disposal, also covering the use and maintenance of the facilities
Food safety	Provision of adequate storage facilities for food (both uncooked and cooked), cooking utensils, adequate quantity of water, and fuel to allow for cooking and reheating
	Provision of information on the importance of food safety
Hand-washing with soap	Provision of soap, allowing for bathing and laundry
	Provision of information on the diseases spread through lack of or poor hand-washing, and demonstration of good hand-washing
Breastfeeding	Provision of information on: the protective qualities of breastfeeding and the importance of breastfeeding sick children
	Practical support to enable mothers to breastfeed sick children

Further reading

Diarrhoea Treatment Guidelines: Including new recommendations for the use of ORS and Zinc supplementation. WHO/UNICEF recommendations, 2004.

The Treatment of diarrhoea: A manual for physicians and other senior health workers. World Health Organization, 2003. (ISBN 92 4 159318 0).

Bahl R et al. Effect of Zinc supplementation on clinical course of acute diarrhoea. Report of a Meeting, New Delhi, 7–8 May 2001. *Journal of Health, Population and Nutrition,* Dec. 2001, Vol. 19(4):338–346.

5.5   Conjunctivitis

Basic facts

- Conjunctivitis is acute inflammation of the conjunctiva of bacterial, viral or allergic origin.
- Bacterial conjunctivitis is cause for most concern in emergency situations.
- Some outbreaks of acute haemorrhagic conjunctivitis due to enterovirus 70 have been observed in refugee populations.
- In areas where trachoma is prevalent, a large proportion of eye disease seen in disaster-affected populations may be due to *Chlamydia trachomatis* infection.
- Conjunctivitis is transmitted by contact with discharges from the conjunctiva of infected people, from contaminated fingers or clothing, and also possibly through mechanical transmission by gnats or flies in some areas.
- Occurrence is widespread throughout the world.
- Epidemics may occur in overcrowded conditions following displacement.

Clinical features

- The clinical course may last from 2 days to 2–3 weeks.
- There is redness, irritation and lacrimation of one or both conjunctiva, followed by oedema of the eyelids and a mucopurulent discharge.

Case management

- Wash both eyes with sterile water or 0.9% saline (or at least with clean boiled water) 4–6 times daily.
- Apply 1% tetracycline eye ointment twice daily for one week.
- Never use topical steroids.

Diagnosis

- Diagnosis is essentially clinical; it does not require microscopic examination of eye discharge in most cases.

Prevention and control measures

- Ensure adequate clean water and soap for personal hygiene and hand-washing.
- Introduce vector control to reduce the fly population if possible.
- Disinfect articles contaminated by conjunctival and nasal discharges.
- In health facilities, ensure vigorous washing of hands by health staff to avoid cross-contamination, and proper disposal of infected material.

5.6 Dengue

Basic facts

- Dengue is an acute febrile viral illness characterized by sudden onset of a fever that lasts for 3–5 days.
- Dengue viruses belong to the family Flaviviridae and include serotypes 1, 2, 3 and 4.
- Transmission occurs through the bite of an infected mosquito (*Aedes aegypti*).
- This mosquito is a daytime-biting species with increased biting 2 hours after sunrise and several hours before sunset.
- The larvae thrive in water in artificial or natural containers close to human habitations, e.g. in old tyres, flower pots, water storage containers or oil drums.
- Recovery from infection with one serotype does not confer protection against the other three serotypes.
- Epidemics are explosive and may affect a high percentage of the population.
- Fatalities in the absence of the more severe dengue haemorrhagic fever are rare.

Clinical features

- Dengue virus infection may be asymptomatic, may cause undifferentiated febrile illness, dengue fever (DF), or dengue haemorrhagic fever (DHF), including dengue shock syndrome (DSS).
- The incubation period is 3–14 days, usually 6–7 days.
- Symptoms include intense headache, myalgia, arthralgia, retro-orbital pain, anorexia and rash.
- Recovery can be associated with prolonged fatigue and depression.
- Children usually have a milder disease than adults.

Diagnosis

- Serum samples are tested for virus-specific antibodies, generally using ELISA techniques. Rapid tests based on dot-blot techniques are commercially available.
- IgM antibody, indicating recent or current infection, is usually detected by day 6–7 after the onset of illness.

Case management

- Supportive treatment should be given – there is no specific therapeutic agent.
- Carefully monitored volume replacement can be life-saving in DHF/DSS.
- There is no available vaccination.
- Contacts should be investigated – determine the place of residence of the patient for the 2 weeks before the onset of illness.

Prevention and control measures

- Eliminate larval habitats of *Aedes* mosquitoes in urban or peri-urban areas.
- Protect against daytime-biting mosquitoes, including the use of screening, protective clothing and repellents.
- Conduct a community survey to determine the density of vector mosquitoes and identify larval habitats.
- In an outbreak, use larvicide on all potential habitats of *Ae. aegypti*.
- Ground applications of ultra-low-volume insecticides can reduce the vector population in an outbreak.
- Carry out social mobilization campaigns to eliminate breeding sites as much as possible.

Further reading

Prevention and control of dengue and dengue haemorrhagic fever: comprehensive guidelines. New Delhi, WHO Regional Office for South-East Asia, 1999 (WHO Regional Publications, South-East Asia Series, No. 29).

Dengue haemorrhagic fever: diagnosis, treatment, prevention and control, 2nd ed. Geneva, World Health Organization, 1997.

5.7　Diphtheria

Basic facts

- Diphtheria is an acute bacterial disease of the tonsils, pharynx, larynx, nose, skin and sometimes the conjunctiva or genitalia.
- It is caused by an aerobic Gram-positive rod, *Corynebacterium diphtheriae*.
- Transmission is by contact (usually direct, rarely indirect) with the respiratory droplets of a patient or carrier, mainly from the nose and throat.
- Case-fatality rates, at 5–10%, have changed little in 50 years.
- A massive outbreak of diphtheria began in the Russian Federation in 1990 and spread to all countries of the former Soviet Union. It was responsible for more than 150 000 reported cases and 5000 deaths. All age groups were affected.
- Vaccine containing diphtheria toxoid (preferably Td) is available and should be given to a population at risk as soon as possible during an epidemic.

Clinical features

- The incubation period is usually 2–5 days, occasionally longer.
- Untreated patients are infectious for 2–3 weeks; antimicrobial treatment usually renders patients non-infectious within 24 hours.
- Classical respiratory diphtheria is characterized by insidious onset and membranous pharyngitis with low-grade fever.

- Although not always present, the membrane is typically grey or white in colour, smooth, thick, fibrinous and firmly adherent.
- It is essential that *all* cases of diphtheria are rapidly identified and properly investigated.
- Diphtheria should be suspected when a patient develops an upper respiratory tract illness with laryngitis or pharyngitis or tonsillitis *plus* adherent membranes of tonsils or nasopharynx.
- A probable case definition is a suspected case plus *one* of the following:
  - recent (< 2 weeks) contact with a confirmed case,
  - diphtheria epidemic currently in the area,
  - stridor,
  - swelling/oedema of the neck,
  - submucosal or skin petechial haemorrhages,
  - toxic circulatory collapse,
  - acute renal insufficiency,
  - myocarditis and/or motor paralysis 1–6 weeks after onset.

Diagnosis

- Throat and nasopharyngeal swabs should be taken *before* antimicrobial treatment is started.

(See Annex 8 for description of sample collection technique.)

Case management

- If diphtheria is strongly suspected, specific treatment with antitoxin and antimicrobial should be initiated immediately.

IMPORTANT: Do not wait for laboratory results before initiating treatment.

- Antitoxin given intramuscularly is the mainstay of treatment: 20 000–100 000 units in a single dose, immediately after throat swabs have been taken.
- Antimicrobial are necessary to eliminate the organism and prevent spread; they are not a substitute for antitoxin treatment.

Management of close contacts

- Close contacts include household members and other persons with a history of direct contact with a diphtheria patient, as well as health care staff exposed to the oral or respiratory secretions of a patient.
- All close contacts should be clinically assessed for symptoms and signs of diphtheria and kept under daily surveillance for 7 days from the last contact.
- Adult contacts must avoid contact with children and must not be allowed to handle food until proven not to be carriers.

- All must receive a single dose of benzathine benzylpenicillin intramuscularly (600 000 units for children under 6 years, 1.2 million units for those 6 years or older). If the culture is positive, antimicrobial should be given as outlined above.
- In an epidemic involving adults, immunize groups that are most affected and at highest risk.

5.8   Hepatitis (viral)

Basic facts

Acute hepatitis (typically presenting as acute jaundice) is generally caused by hepatitis A, B, C and E viruses, which belong to different virus families. These viruses also differ in their (*a*) modes of transmission, (*b*) geographical and epidemiological patterns, which explain various age-related incidence profiles, and (*c*) propensity to result or not in chronic infections. Hepatitis D (not detailed any further here) is a particular case, being caused by a defective virus that can replicate and cause disease only in individuals already co-infected or chronically infected with the hepatitis B virus.

Table 5.5 illustrates the main differences between the hepatitis viruses.

Table 5.5   **Characteristics of the hepatitis viruses**

Virus	Family	Transmission	Main groups at risk of infection	Complications
Hepatitis A	Picornaviridae	Faecal–oral	Non-immune travellers to regions where sanitation is problematic (in low endemicity areas) Young children, usually asymptomatic (in high-endemicity areas)	Fulminant hepatitis
Hepatitis B	Hepadnaviridae	Parenteral + sexual	Injecting drugs users Contact with infected blood or blood products High-risk sexual behaviour	Fulminant hepatitis Chronic hepatitis, cirrhosis, liver cancer
Hepatitis C	Flaviviridae	Parenteral (+/− sexual)	Injection drugs users Contact with infected blood or blood products	Fulminant hepatitis Chronic hepatitis, cirrhosis, liver cancer
Hepatitis E	Currently unclassified	Faecal–oral	Large outbreaks in communities with inadequate water/waste water facilities Non-immune travellers to regions where HEV is endemic (very rare)	Fulminant hepatitis Mortality up to 20% in pregnancy

Cases of viral hepatitis are seen all over the world, occurring either sporadically or during epidemics of various magnitudes. Outbreaks of hepatitis A and hepatitis E have been documented in refugee and internally displaced person camps (Chad, Kenya, Kosovo, Namibia, Sudan).

This can be explained by the specific patterns of transmission of viral hepatitis.

✔ Hepatitis A virus transmitted by the faecal–oral route is already highly prevalent in countries with poor sanitary infrastructure. Under such circumstances, transmission generally occurs during childhood, at an age when most of the infections due to these viruses are mild or generally asymptomatic. This leaves the bulk of adult populations largely immune to new infections, and therefore protected against the most severe forms of the diseases typically seen at older ages. Hepatitis E has been found confined to geographical areas where faecal contamination of drinking-water is common. Most outbreaks have occurred following monsoon rains, heavy flooding, contamination of well water, or massive uptake of untreated sewage into city water-treatment plants. Further disruption of social and health infrastructures during emergencies in developing countries is expected at most to increase transmission of hepatitis A and E. Only when disasters hit populations previously enjoying good standards of sanitation, or countries with transition economies, is there a theoretically increased risk of outbreaks of hepatitis A or E.

✔ Transmission of hepatitis B and hepatitis C could potentially be of concern during emergencies under circumstances favouring the increased use of unsafe injection practices, illicit injecting drug use, unsafe sexual activities, or the use of unreliable blood transfusion facilities. Transmission of hepatitis among specific groups at risk under such circumstances is unlikely to be detected during the acute phase of an emergency, but should be taken into consideration in the planning of preventive activities and in the design of an integrated health surveillance system.

Clinical features

Depending on the age at infection, the type of virus, and other (generally unknown) factors, viral hepatitis can lead to:

• asymptomatic infection,

• acute uncomplicated jaundice,

• fulminant hepatitis.

(Chronic infection is not relevant in the situation of an emergency.)

Diagnosis

• Sporadic cases of acute jaundice with no or moderate fever are generally due to acute viral hepatitis, especially in young adults. Careful clinical examination should detect other causes of jaundice possibly requiring specific treatment (e.g. surgery and antimicrobial therapy for obstructive jaundice). Clusters of cases of acute jaundice should lead to epidemiological investigations to exclude transmissible diseases with important public health implications (yellow fever, leptospirosis, etc.).

- Routine laboratory techniques to confirm the diagnosis of acute hepatitis and its etiology are not always available in emergency situations. When an outbreak is suspected, serum samples should be sent to a reference laboratory for determination of the causative organism.

- Serodiagnostic tests are available to screen potential blood donors for hepatitis B and C (and HIV) infection. Rapid tests that do not require specific laboratory equipment are being developed for the detection of serological markers.

Case management

- Acute uncomplicated viral hepatitis simply requires supportive therapy.

- Acute fulminant hepatitis carries a poor prognosis and requires intensive treatment capacities that are generally beyond the technical possibilities available in emergencies.

- Barrier nursing should be carried out of patients presenting with acute jaundice of possibly infectious origin.

- Acute hepatitis in pregnant women (particularly during the last trimester) requires careful monitoring, as hepatitis E constitutes a major risk of death from complications of pregnancy (including spontaneous death of the embryo) or of fulminant hepatitis.

Prevention and control measures

- Control and prevention of hepatitis A or E require the enforcement of water and food sanitation (see Chapter 2).

- Control and prevention of hepatitis B and C require safe injection practices (see Section 2.6.2). Where blood transfusion services are provided, screening of all blood products is mandatory for hepatitis B and C and HIV.

- Vaccines are available that protect against hepatitis A and B for several years. There is no indication for mass vaccination against hepatitis B in emergencies. In the case of an outbreak of hepatitis A, targeted vaccination of population groups at risk is recommended. Health workers should be immune to hepatitis B owing to previous vaccination. Systematic vaccination might be considered for health workers expected not to be immune to hepatitis A and B, and those exposed to particular risks owing to the emergency.

5.9 HIV/AIDS

Basic facts

- Acquired immunodeficiency syndrome (AIDS) is the late clinical stage of infection with the human immunodeficiency virus (HIV).
- Sub-Saharan Africa accounts for more than 60% of all people living with HIV, yet the region has just over 10% of the world's population.
- In 2004, an estimated 4.9 million people globally became newly infected, while 3.1 million died of AIDS.
- At the end of 2004, an estimated 39.4 million people were living with HIV globally.
- Women and girls make up almost 57% of adults living with HIV in sub-Saharan Africa.
- There are four main modes of transmission of HIV:
  - sexual intercourse (vaginal or anal) with an infected partner, especially in the presence of a concurrent ulcerative or non-ulcerative sexually transmitted infection (STI);
  - contaminated needles (injecting drug use, needlestick injuries, injections);
  - transfusion of infected blood or blood products;
  - mother-to-child transmission during pregnancy, labour and delivery or through breastfeeding.

(The main risk factors for increased HIV transmission in emergencies are shown in Table 5.6.)

Clinical features

- The incubation time is variable. On average, the time from HIV infection to the development of clinical AIDS is eight to ten years, though AIDS may be manifested in less than two years or be delayed in onset beyond ten years.
- Incubation times are shortened in resource-poor settings and in older patients. They can be prolonged by provision of primary prophylaxis for opportunistic infections or antiretroviral treatment.
- Infected people may then be free of clinical signs or symptoms for many months to years.
- Infectiousness is observed to be high during the initial period after infection. Studies suggest it increases further with increasing immune deficiency, clinical symptoms and the presence of other STIs.
- The severity of HIV-related opportunistic infection is correlated with the degree of immune system dysfunction.

Modified 1985 WHO case definition for AIDS surveillance (the "Bangui definition") [a,b]

An adult or adolescent (> 12 years of age) is considered to have AIDS if at least two of the following major signs are present in combination with at least one of the minor signs listed below, and if these signs are not known to be due to a condition unrelated to HIV infection.

Major signs

- Weight loss >10% of body weight
- Chronic diarrhoea for >1 month
- Prolonged fever for >1 month (intermittent or constant)

Minor signs

- Persistent cough for >1 month [c]
- Generalized pruritic dermatitis
- History of herpes zoster
- Oropharyngeal candidiasis
- Chronic progressive or disseminated herpes simplex infection
- Generalized lymphadenopathy

The presence of either generalized Kaposi sarcoma or cryptococcal meningitis is sufficient for the diagnosis of AIDS for surveillance purposes.

[a] Source: *Weekly Epidemiological Record*, 1994, **69**:273–275.
[b] Clinical under review: see *Interim WHO clinical staging of HIV/AIDS and HIV/AIDS-case definitions for surveillance* (document WHO/HIV/2005.02).
[c] For patients with tuberculosis, persistent cough for more than a month should not be considered a minor sign.

Table 5.6   **Risk factors for increased HIV transmission in emergencies**

Population movement

- In emergency situations, population movement often causes breakdown in family and social ties, and erodes traditional values and coping strategies. This can result in higher-risk sexual behaviour, which increases the risk of the spread of HIV.
- In high-incidence regions, refugees from areas where HIV is uncommon may find themselves exposed to a higher HIV risk, which, together with little prior knowledge of HIV risks and prevention, will increase their vulnerability to infection.

Overcrowding

- Groups with differing levels of HIV awareness, and differing rates of infection, are often placed together in temporary locations such as refugee camps, where there is a greater than normal potential for sexual contact.

Poor access to health services

- Without adequate medical services STIs, if left untreated in either partner, greatly increase the risk of

acquiring HIV.
- Important materials for HIV prevention, particularly condoms, are likely to be lacking in an emergency situation.

Sexual violence
- Refugees and internally displaced persons are often physically and socially powerless, with women and children at particular risk of sexual coercion, abuse or rape.
- Sexual violence carries a higher risk of infection because the person violated cannot protect herself or himself from unsafe sex, and because the virus can be transmitted more easily if body tissues are torn during violent sex.

Sex work
- Exchange of sexual favours for basic needs, such as money, shelter, security, etc., is common in or around refugee camps, and inevitably involves both the refugee and the host community. Both sex workers and clients are at risk of HIV infection if unprotected sex is practised.

Injecting drug use
- In the typical conditions of an emergency, it is highly likely that drug injectors will be sharing needles, a practice that carries a very high risk of HIV transmission if one of the people sharing is infected.

Unsafe blood transfusions
- Transfusion with HIV-infected blood is a highly efficient means of transmitting the virus. In emergency situations, when regular transfusion services have broken down, it is particularly difficult to ensure blood safety.

Adolescent health
- Children in refugee settings may have little to occupy themselves, which may lead them to experiment with sex earlier than children in other situations.

1994 expanded WHO case definition for AIDS surveillance (to be used where HIV serological testing is available)

An adult or adolescent (>12 years of age) is considered to have AIDS if a test for HIV antibody gives a positive result, and one or more of the following conditions are present:
- a greater than 10% body weight loss or cachexia, with diarrhoea or fever or both, intermittent or constant, for at least 1 month, not known to be due to a condition unrelated to HIV;
- cryptococcal meningitis;
- pulmonary or extrapulmonary tuberculosis;
- Kaposi sarcoma;
- neurological impairment sufficient to prevent independent daily activities, not known to be due to a condition unrelated to HIV infection (e.g. trauma or cerebro-vascular accident);
- candidiasis of the oesophagus (which may be presumptively diagnosed based on the presence of oral candidiasis accompanied by dysphagia);
- clinically diagnosed life-threatening or recurrent episodes of pneumonia, with or without etiological confirmation;

- invasive cervical cancer.

Diagnosis

- This is most commonly done by detecting HIV antibody in serum samples using enzyme-linked immunoassay (ELISA or EIA). When this test is positive, it must be confirmed with another test of higher specificity such as the Western blot, the indirect fluorescent antibody (IFA) test or a second ELISA test that is methodologically and/or antigenically independent.
- The rapid tests, which are recommended by WHO, have been evaluated at WHO collaborating centres and have levels of sensitivity and specificity comparable to WHO-recommended ELISA tests. The use of rapid HIV tests may afford several advantages in emergency and disaster settings.
  - Rapid tests that do not require refrigeration will be more suitable for remote and rural areas and sites without a guaranteed electricity supply. Long shelf life is also important, especially for remote areas and sites performing smaller numbers of tests.
  - Many rapid tests require no laboratory equipment and can be performed in settings where electricity and water supplies need not be guaranteed.
  - Rapid tests can detect HIV antibodies in whole blood (finger prick samples) as well as serum/plasma, and testing may therefore be performed by non-laboratory personnel with adequate training and supervision.
  - Rapid tests reduce the incidence of persons failing to obtain test results. In emergency situations persons may be relocated frequently and therefore not obtain their results.
  - The WHO bulk purchasing scheme has reduced the price of rapid HIV tests to between US$ 0.42 and US$ 2 per test. Rapid tests are slightly more expensive than ELISA tests, but since ELISA tests are multiple tests, the cost per test is in practice considerably higher unless all reagent wells (40–90) are used.
- ELISA tests were originally developed for blood screening and these assays are suitable for batch testing (testing at least 40–90 specimens per run). ELISA tests are suitable for large *voluntary counselling and testing* (VCT) settings, but in many VCT sites the ability to perform single tests or small numbers of tests is an advantage.

Case management

- Provide high-quality care and support to all people living with HIV/AIDS that includes counselling, psychosocial support, treatment for opportunistic infections (e.g. tuberculosis), palliative care and access to antiretroviral therapy where feasible.

- Support people living with HIV/AIDS to live normal and productive lives that are free of stigmatization and discrimination.

Prevention and control measures (see Table 5.7)

Table 5.7 **Prevention and control measures to reduce HIV transmission in emergency situations**

Reduce sexual and mother-to-child transmission
- Awareness and life skills education, especially for young people, to ensure that all people are well informed of what does and does not constitute a mode of transmission; of how and where to acquire free condoms and medical attention if necessary; and of basic hygiene.
- Condom promotion, which would ensure that good quality condoms are freely available to those who need them, together with culturally sensitive instructions and distribution.
- STI control, including for sex workers, using the syndromic STI management approach (as laboratory services for confirmation are unlikely to be available in emergencies), with partner notification and promotion of safer sex.
- Reduction of mother-to-child transmission of HIV by:
  - the primary prevention of HIV among women, especially young women;
  - avoiding unintended pregnancies among HIV-infected women and promoting family planning methods, particularly in women who are infected with HIV;
  - preventing the transmission of HIV from infected pregnant women to their infants by:
    - using an antiretroviral prophylaxis regimen,
    - avoiding unnecessary invasive obstetrical procedures, such as artificial rupture of membranes or episiotomy,
    - modifying infant feeding practices (replacement feeding given with a cup when acceptable, feasible, affordable, sustainable and safe, otherwise exclusive breastfeeding for the first months of life is recommended).

Blood safety
- HIV testing of all transfused blood.
- Avoidance of non-essential blood transfusion.
- Recruitment of safe blood donor pool.

Universal precautions
- Washing hands thoroughly with soap and water, especially after contact with body fluids or wounds.
- Using protective gloves and clothing when there is risk of contact with blood or other potentially infected body fluids.
- Safe handling and disposing of waste material, needles and other sharp instruments. Properly cleaning and disinfecting medical instruments between patients.

Physical protection
- Protecting the most vulnerable, especially women and children, from violence and abuse is not only an important principle of human rights but also essential for reducing the risk of HIV infection.

Protecting health care workers
- To reduce nosocomial transmission, health workers should strictly adhere to the universal precautions with all patients and laboratory samples, whether or not known to be infected with HIV.
- Health care workers should have access to voluntary counselling, testing and care. Often health workers deployed in complex emergencies experience significant occupational stress, and those tested as part of the management of occupational exposures will require additional support.

- Post-exposure prophylaxis (PEP) kits must be made available to protect humanitarian workers who have been sexually assaulted. PEP kits should include emergency contraception and double/triple anti-retroviral treatment. PEP kits are distributed through the United Nations dispensary system.

Counselling and voluntary testing programmes

- In the acute emergency, it is important that available resources for HIV testing should be devoted to ensuring a safe blood supply for transfusions.
- The establishment of voluntary testing and counselling services to help individuals make informed decisions on HIV testing should be considered when relative stability is restored. Often refugees are coerced into testing, or are required to make a decision with regard to testing, when they are suffering acute or post-traumatic stress disorders.
- As refugees are often tested before resettlement in other countries, it is critical that they receive counselling on the legal and social implications of the test. Often migration or temporary residency status is contingent on the applicant being seronegative.
- Post-test counselling is essential for both seronegative and seropositive results. Refugees and conflict survivors who are already traumatized will require additional psychosocial support if they test sero-positive. Typically the support networks of displaced persons are disrupted, and suicide risk assessment forms an important part of post-test counselling in a refugee or conflict context.
- Testing of orphaned minors should be done, with the consent of their official guardians, only where there is an immediate health concern or benefit to the child. There should be no mandatory screening before admittance to substitute care.

Vaccination

- Asymptomatic HIV-infected children should be immunized with EPI vaccines.
- Symptomatic HIV-infected children should *not* receive BCG or yellow fever vaccine.

Further reading

UNAIDS report summaries in *UNAIDS December 2004 epidemic update* at: http://www.unaids.org/wad2004/report_pdf.html

Guidelines for HIV Interventions in Emergency Settings, 2004. UN Interagency Standing Committee (IASC), Taskforce on HIV/AIDS in Emergency Settings.

Migrant populations and HIV/AIDS: the development and implementation of programmes: theory, methodology and practice. Geneva, Joint United Nations Programme on HIV/AIDS, 2000 (UNAIDS Best Practice Collection – Key Material).

5.10 Japanese encephalitis

Basic facts

- Japanese encephalitis (JE) is an acute inflammatory disease caused by a flavivirus, involving the brain, spinal cord and meninges.
- Less than 1% of human infections are clinically apparent, but the case-fatality rate among persons with clinical disease is 25–50%.
- Infants and elderly people are most susceptible to severe disease.
- The disease occurs in eastern, south-eastern and southern Asia.
- the disease is especially associated with rice-growing areas.

- Transmission is through the bite of an infected mosquito of species commonly found in rice fields. *Culex tritaeniorhynchus* is the most common, but other *Culex* species including *Cx. annulirostris*, *Cx. vishnui* complex and *Cx. gelidus* may be involved locally).
- The reservoirs of the virus are pigs and some species of wild bird (especially herons and egrets).

Clinical features

- The incubation period is usually 5–15 days.
- Symptoms can include: headache, fever, meningeal signs, stupor, disorientation, coma, tremors, paresis (generalized), hypertonia, loss of coordination. The encephalitis cannot be distinguished clinically from other central nervous system infections.
- Severe infections are marked by acute onset, headache, high fever, meningeal signs and coma.
- JE infections are common and the majority are asymptomatic. They may occur concurrently with other infections causing central nervous system symptoms, and serological evidence of recent JE viral infection may not be correct in indicating JE to be the cause of the illness.

Diagnosis

- Diagnosis is by demonstration of specific IgM in acute-phase serum or cerebrospinal fluid.

Case management

- Supportive treatment should be given – there is no specific therapeutic agent.
- Contacts should be investigated – determine the place of residence of the patient for the two weeks before the onset of illness.

Prevention and control measures

- Avoid exposure to mosquitoes and use protective clothing and repellents.
- Screen sleeping and living quarters.
- House pigs away from living quarters.
- Japanese encephalitis vaccines are available for travellers to endemic areas, and systematic human mass vaccination has probably contributed significantly to the declining incidence in several endemic countries.
- Vaccination of pigs and fogging with insecticide from aircraft have proved effective as control measures during outbreaks, but both methods of control are very expensive.

Further reading

Thongcharoen P. Japanese encephalitis virus encephalitis: an overview. *Southeast Asian Journal of Tropical Medicine and Public Health,* 1989, **20**:559–573.

Igarashi A. Epidemiology and control of Japanese encephalitis. *World Health Statistics Quarterly*, 1992, **45**:299–305.

5.11 Leishmaniasis

Basic facts

- The causal agents are *Leishmania* spp., protozoa transmitted by the bite of sandflies. Some 30 species of sandfly are proven vectors; the usual reservoir hosts are domestic and/or wild animals (zoonotic leishmaniasis). In some cases, humans are the sole reservoir hosts (anthroponotic leishmaniasis).

- The main clinical forms of the disease are: visceral leishmaniasis (*kala azar*), localized cutaneous leishmaniasis and (mainly in the western hemisphere) mucocutaneous leishmaniasis. Table 5.8 sets out the reservoirs of these three forms.

Table 5.8   **Reservoirs of leishmaniasis**

Form	Animal reservoir (zoonotic forms)	Human reservoir (anthroponotic forms)
Visceral leishmaniasis (VL)	Dogs	Epidemic situations or HIV co-infection
Cutaneous leishmaniasis (CL)	Rodents (rural foci)	Urban foci
Mucocutaneous leishmaniasis (MCL)	Sylvatic mammals	Not applicable

- The leishmaniases are currently prevalent on all continents except Australia and Antarctica, and are considered to be endemic in 88 countries, 72 of which are developing countries:
  - 90% of visceral leishmaniasis cases occur in Bangladesh, Brazil, India, Nepal and Sudan;
  - 90% of mucocutaneous leishmaniasis cases occur in Bolivia, Brazil and Peru;
  - 90% of cutaneous leishmaniasis cases occur in Afghanistan, Brazil, Iran, Peru, Saudi Arabia and Syria.
- The incubation period varies from weeks to months.
- Epidemics are linked to human migrations from rural to poor suburban areas; in zoonotic foci, epidemics are related to environmental changes and movement of non-immune people to rural areas. There have been severe epidemics of visceral leishmaniasis among refugees and internally displaced persons in recent years, notably in Sudan. Anthroponotic cutaneous

leishmaniasis reaches epidemic proportions in Afghanistan, the most important focus in the world being in the capital, Kabul.

Clinical features

- Cutaneous leishmaniasis is characterized by the appearance of one or more skin lesions, typically on uncovered parts of the body (face, neck, arms and legs). A nodule may appear at the site of inoculation and may enlarge to become an indolent ulcer. The sore remains in this stage for a variable time before healing, typically leaving a depressed permanent scar. Other atypical forms may occur.

- In some individuals, certain strains of mucocutaneous leishmaniasis can disseminate and cause extensive and disfiguring mucosal lesions of the nose, mouth and throat cavities.

- Visceral leishmaniasis is characterized by prolonged irregular fever, spleno-megaly, hepatomegaly, anaemia and weight loss. It is usually fatal if untreated.

Diagnosis

- The diagnosis of cutaneous leishmaniasis is essentially clinical but may require a stained smear in atypical cases; no serological test is available.

- The diagnosis of mucocutaneous leishmaniasis is clinical, but may require stained smear in atypical cases. Serological tests are also available.

- In the case of visceral leishmaniasis, splenic aspiration is the most sensitive technique but exposes the patient to frequent complications (sometimes lethal). The procedure requires preliminary confirmation of normal coagulation tests, and the availability of blood transfusion and emergency surgery services should complications occur. Such precautions make the procedure unsuitable for routine use in district hospitals in endemic areas and in most emergency situations. A rapid and sensitive serological test, the direct agglutination test, is available. It is recommended as the basis of test–treatment strategies for visceral leishmaniasis in areas where the disease is endemic.

Case management

Current treatments are based on pentavalent antimonials as first-line drugs. In the presence of resistance the use of second-line drugs is possible (amphotericin B, aminosidine plus pentavalent antimonials or pentamidine isethionate) but these are unlikely to be available and/or affordable in emergency situations.

Most cases of cutaneous leishmaniasis can be treated by intralesional injections of pentavalent antimony. Visceral leishmaniasis, mucocutaneous leishmaniasis and multilesional or severe forms of cutaneous leishmaniasis require long courses of parenteral injections of first- or second-line drugs.

Resistance of visceral leishmaniasis to pentavalent antimony treatment is widespread in north-eastern India.

Leishmania/**HIV co-infection**

AIDS and other immunosuppressive conditions increase the risk of *Leishmania*-infected people developing visceral illness. Leishmaniasis accelerates the onset of AIDS by cumulative immunosuppression and by stimulating the replication of the virus.

Leishmania/HIV co-infections have already been reported from over 30 countries, and the extension of the geographical overlap of visceral leishmaniasis and AIDS is on the increase.

The risk of transmission of visceral leishmaniasis is increasing through the sharing of infected needles by intravenous drug users.

Prevention and control measures

See Table 5.9.

Table 5.9   **Control measures for leishmaniasis**

Measure	Visceral leishmaniasis		Cutaneous leishmaniasis		Mucocutaneous leishmaniasis
	Anthroponotic	Zoonotic	Anthroponotic	Zoonotic	Zoonotic
Reinforced surveillance, early detection and treatment	Priority intervention				
Reduction of animal reservoirs	Not applicable	Large-scale screening, followed by killing of infected dogs in emergency situations	Not applicable	To be adapted to each particular species of animal reservoir	Not feasible owing to ecology of animal reservoirs
Vector control	Residual insecticide house spraying recommended in severe epidemic situations	Residual insecticide spraying of houses and animal shelters recommended in severe epidemic situations	Residual insecticide house spraying recommended in severe epidemic situations	Environmental management	Environmental management
Individual protection against vector: insecticide impregnated bednets	Essential in epidemic situations			Not recommended	Not recommended
Health promotion/ social mobilization	Essential in epidemic situations				

Further reading

Manual on visceral leishmaniasis control. Geneva, World Health Organization, 1996 (document WHO/LEISH/96.40).

WHO report on global surveillance of epidemic-prone infectious diseases. Chapter 10. Leishmaniasis and Leishmania/HIV co-infection. Geneva, World Health Organization, 2000 (document WHO/CDS/CSR/ISR/2000.1).

5.12 Malaria

Basic facts

- Malaria is a parasitic disease caused by protozoan parasites of the genus *Plasmodium*.

- Only four plasmodium species develop in humans: *P. falciparum* (causing the life-threatening form of malaria), *P. vivax, P. ovale and P. malariae*. Of these, only *P. vivax* and *P. ovale* have persistent liver forms that may lead to relapses after the initial blood infection has been cured.

- *P. falciparum* and *P. vivax* are the main species of public health importance. *P. falciparum* is the commonest species throughout the tropics and sub-tropics – up to 80–90% of malaria cases in sub-Saharan African countries are due to *P. falciparum*.

- The disease is transmitted from person to person by *Anopheles* mosquitoes, which mainly bite between dusk and dawn.

- In the blood, parasites develop asexual (trophozoite) and sexual (gametocyte) forms, which are responsible for clinical attacks and disease transmission, respectively.

- Malaria parasites can also be transmitted by transfusion of blood from an infected to a healthy person and occasionally from mother to fetus.

- Almost 300 million malaria cases occur every year with more than 1 million deaths, 90% of which (according to WHO estimates) occur in African countries, south of the Sahara.

Natural history

- Depending on temperature and humidity, the average development period in the mosquito is 12 days for *P. falciparum*, 13–17 days for *P. ovale and P. vivax* (but in some strains up to 9 months) and 28–30 days for *P. malariae*.

- The incubation period in humans is the time between the infective bite and the first appearance of clinical signs, of which fever is the most common. It varies according to *Plasmodium* species, being the shortest for *P. falciparum* (9–13 days) and the longest for *P. malariae* (years).

- The minimum period of time between the initial infection of the mosquito and the development of clinical symptoms in humans is 3–4 weeks.

Clinical case definitions

- In *uncomplicated malaria*, the patient presents with fever or history of fever within the last 48 hours (with or without other symptoms such as nausea, vomiting and diarrhoea, headache, back pain, chills and myalgia).

- In a *high malaria risk* area or season, children with fever and no general danger sign or stiff neck should be classified as having malaria. Although a substantial number of children will be treated for malaria when in fact they have another febrile illness, presumptive treatment for malaria is justified in this category given the high rate of malaria risk and the possibility that another illness might cause the malaria infection to progress.

- In a *low malarial risk area* or season, children with fever (or history of fever) and no general danger sign or stiff neck are classified as having malaria, and given an antimalarial only if they have no runny nose (a sign of ARI), no measles, and no other obvious cause of fever (pneumonia, sore throat, etc.).

- In *severe malaria*, patients present with symptoms as for uncomplicated malaria, and also drowsiness with extreme weakness and associated signs and symptoms related to organ failure, such as disorientation, loss of consciousness, convulsions, severe anaemia, jaundice, haemoglobinuria, spontaneous bleeding, pulmonary oedema and shock.

Diagnosis

- Laboratory diagnosis is by demonstration of malaria parasites in a blood film (thick or thin smear). Rapid diagnostic tests are useful but can be user-dependent and spurious if stored at > 30°.

- In highly endemic areas of Africa, people gradually develop immunity to the disease and parasitaemia may occur without clinical symptoms, especially in adults. In these situations, the clinical picture is used to guide treatment decisions. In non-immune populations and less endemic areas, all parasitaemias may lead to clinical disease and should be treated.

- Laboratory diagnosis may not be possible in the acute phase of an emergency where laboratory services are unavailable. In this situation, diagnosis must depend on clinical symptoms combined with knowledge of the risk of malaria. This is generally not very accurate, and an attempt should be made to at least define the percentage of malaria patients among all those with fever. Rapid diagnostic tests can be useful, particularly in emergency settings.

- The relatively high cost of rapid diagnostic tests may be justified in areas where drug resistance necessitates the use of newer, more expensive antimalarial drugs.

- Microscopic diagnosis is essential for the management of suspected treatment failures, especially in areas where *P. vivax* and drug-resistant *P. falciparum* occur simultaneously.

Treatment

Plasmodium falciparum

Treatment policy should be based on knowledge of drug resistance patterns in the area. This is particularly important as displaced populations are especially vulnerable owing to low immunity (from malnutrition or lack of previous exposure to malaria) and to the risk of being unable to seek re-treatment if treatment fails.

Local, up-to-date information on drug resistance is essential for developing an appropriate treatment policy. Local health authorities, which may have the information already, and operational agencies should collaborate in obtaining the information. Other causes of treatment failure, such as non-compliance, vomiting and poor-quality drugs, should always be monitored. Drug efficacy monitoring should follow standard procedures as developed by WHO.[3] As drug resistance is rapidly developing, it is also important to evaluate second-line or future treatments prospectively. The first-line treatment may need to be changed if drug resistance studies show that the national policy is ineffective (i.e. with 15% resistance to therapy).

Combinations of artemisinin derivatives (such as artesunate, artemether, dihydroartemisinin) and various other antimalarials are increasingly being used as first-line treatment policy.[4] Artemisinin-based combination therapy (ACT) has distinct advantages: the artemisinins produce rapid clinical and parasitological cure; there is as yet no documented parasite resistance to them; they reduce the gametocyte carrier rate and thus reduce transmission; and they are generally well tolerated. This option includes, for instance, artesunate plus amodiaquine, artesunate plus sulfadoxine–pyrimethamine (SP) and artemether–lumefantrine (Coartem®). A drawback of artemisinins is the limited data on safety in pregnancy. Artemisinin compounds are not recommended in the first trimester of pregnancy and currently quinine is used as an alternative. ACT may be used in the second or third trimester of pregnancy if there is no better alternative. The lack of data for the use of the 6-dose regimen of Coartem® under 10 kg body weight currently limits its use in small children who should be treated with quinine.

The details of the management of severe falciparum malaria are discussed elsewhere.[5] The use of daily intramuscular artemether is operationally preferable to 8–12-hourly quinine administration for the management of severe malaria in emergencies and other situations with limited nursing care.

---

[3] *Monitoring antimalarial drug resistance*. Geneva, World Health Organization, 2002 (document WHO/CDS/RBM/2002.39).

[4] *The use of antimalarial drugs*. Geneva, World Health Organization, 2001 (document WHO/CDS/RBM/2001.33).

[5] *Management of severe malaria – a practical handbook*, 2nd ed. Geneva, World Health Organization, 2000.

Plasmodium vivax

Chloroquine is the treatment of choice in areas where *only P. vivax* occurs. Owing to compliance and operational constraints, wide-scale use of 14-day primaquine anti-relapse treatment is usually not feasible in emergency situations. Anti-relapse treatment is not useful for patients living in endemic areas with unabated transmission.

Where *P. falciparum* and *P. vivax* co-exist and microscopy is not available, *P. vivax* generally responds well to the drugs used for *P. falciparum*. The exception is SP, which is not suitable for treatment of *P. vivax*. Thus, in countries such as Timor-Leste, where there is a relatively high percentage of *P. vivax* infections among malaria cases and where *P. falciparum* has become increasingly resistant to chloroquine, the first-line policy for clinically diagnosed cases is now a combination of SP (against *P. falciparum*) plus chloroquine (against *P. vivax*). These policies stipulate that patients with microscopically confirmed malaria receive either chloroquine or SP, depending on the species identified. Localized *P. vivax* resistance to chloroquine has been reported from several countries in Asia and the Americas.

Chemoprophylaxis and intermittent preventive treatment

Malaria chemoprophylaxis is essential for non-immune expatriate staff working in camps and communities in *P. falciparum*-endemic areas. It should be combined with rigorous protection against mosquito bites. The choice of drugs is between chloroquine + proguanil, mefloquine, doxycycline and atovaquone-proguanil. In *P. vivax*-only areas, chloroquine prophylaxis may be used to prevent malaria. The recommended prophylaxis regimen varies by area; details are available in *International travel and health* at *http://www.who.int/ith*.

In highly endemic *P. falciparum* areas, where malaria in pregnancy is associated with high maternal and infant morbidity and mortality, semi-immune primigravidae and secundigravidae (first and second pregnancies) should receive intermittent preventive treatment (IPT) with an effective (preferably single-dose, such as SP) antimalarial drug delivered in the context of antenatal care. Such intermittent preventive treatment should be started from the second trimester onwards. IPT doses should not be given more frequently than monthly.

All pregnant women should receive at least 2 doses of IPT after quickening (onset of fetal movements), during routinely scheduled antenatal clinic visits as recommended by WHO (4 antenatal visits, with 3 visits after quickening). There is no evidence that receiving 3 or more doses of IPT with SP will result in an increased risk of adverse drug reactions. Studies indicate that HIV-positive pregnant women may need such intermittent preventive treatment on a monthly basis during all pregnancies to achieve optimal benefit. To achieve optimal benefit in settings with HIV prevalence in pregnant women of greater than 12%, it is more cost-effective to treat all women with 3 or more doses of

IPT with SP, instead of screening for HIV and providing this regimen only to HIV-positive women.

In areas of unstable malaria transmission, women of reproductive age have relatively little acquired immunity to malaria, and hence all pregnant women are at similar risk for malaria infection. Its consequences in these settings are maternal illness, severe malaria with central nervous system complications, anaemia, and adverse reproductive outcomes, including stillbirths, abortions, and low birth weight. Abortion is common in the first trimester, and prematurity is common in third trimester. Other consequences during pregnancy commonly associated with *P. falciparum* infection include hypoglycaemia, hyperpyrexia, severe haemolytic anaemia, and pulmonary oedema.

The effects during pregnancy of the other three parasites that cause malaria in humans (*P. vivax, P. malariae,* and *P. ovale*) are less clear. In these areas, *P. vivax* infections are likely to result in febrile illness. A study among non-immune pregnant women in Thailand reported that *P. vivax* malaria during pregnancy is associated with maternal anaemia and low birth weight, but to a lesser extent than *P. falciparum*. There is also a need to assess whether antimalarial prophylaxis with chloroquine may be justified in areas where *P. vivax* infection among pregnant women is common and contributes to maternal anaemia and infant low birth weight.

Prevention and control measures

The main methods of preventing malaria and reducing transmission in emergency situations are (specific indications are detailed in vector control strategies in Section 2.4.2):

- Rapid diagnosis and effective case management – important in reducing malaria transmission.
- Insecticide-treated mosquito nets (ITN) – where the population is sensitized and shelters are appropriate for hanging nets.
- Permethrin-sprayed blankets, sheets and chaddors (proven efficacy in Asia and undergoing field trials in Africa under highly endemic conditions).
- Permethrin-treated outer clothing worn in the evening or in bed (effective in south Asia).
- Indoor residual spraying of insecticide ("house spraying") – the method of control most often used in emergency situations.
- Environmental control – difficult during the acute phase except on a local scale, and impact is often limited.
- Insecticide-treated plastic sheeting – is currently undergoing field trials.

Malaria outbreak

In a suspected *P. falciparum* malaria outbreak, there may be a need to deviate from national treatment protocols if the first-line treatment is shown to be ineffective. WHO recommends the use of an efficacious (100%), safe, acceptable regimen that allows good compliance.

For uncomplicated malaria, ACT is currently the only treatment that fits this recommendation except in some regions (such as Central America) where there are strong data on the high efficacy of other drugs. Where ACT is not used, primaquine as a single-dose gametocidal should be used to reduce transmission. In pregnant women, ACT is contraindicated in the first trimester; it may be used in the second or third trimester if there is no better alternative.

For severe malaria, the guiding principle for choice of drugs in an outbreak should be to use an efficacious, safe drug (minor side-effects are tolerable) that reduces staff workload and does not require complicated infrastructure. Intramuscular artemether is the drug of choice as it has similar efficacy to quinine but has lower requirements for monitoring. Artesunate suppositories may be used as pre-referral medication. If the patient cannot be transferred, rectal artesunate can be continued until oral intake is established.

In a pure *P. vivax* outbreak, chloroquine should be the first-line therapy. Anti-relapse therapy with primaquine is unnecessary during an outbreak. The minimal information required to reduce mortality is presented in Table 5.10.

Deciding on the intervention to adopt will depend on available resources, the capacity of the health system and other health priorities. The main aim of the response is to reduce mortality and disease burden. Three strategies for case management are feasible depending on the situation:

* mass treatment of fever cases in absence of rapid diagnostic tests,
* active case detection through mobile outreach services,
* passive case detection.

In a severe outbreak, the majority of fever cases may be due to malaria. Even if microscopy is available there may not be time to confirm the diagnosis of every suspected case. Rapid diagnostic tests are very useful in these situations, although a negative test does not preclude treatment. In the absence of these tests, mass treatment of febrile cases is then justified. Microscopy is, however, very useful for monitoring epidemic trends through the monitoring of slide positivity rates (i.e. malaria as a proportion of all febrile illness) in samples of slides taken from fever cases at regular intervals.

Health services should reach as deeply into the community as possible and make full use of community health workers if available. **Active** detection of malaria cases in the community is justified during an outbreak if excess mortality is documented, the population is dispersed, there is a lack of health facilities and referral systems are unavailable. Again, rapid diagnostic tests can be very useful for case detection. Ideally, treatments should be efficacious, short and simple to avoid the necessity for follow-up or the chances of severe malaria developing. Outreach clinics should include a health education component and ideally should be equipped to manage severe cases.

Clinic-based **passive** case detection is more suited to chronic situations once mortality is under control. Laboratory services with quality control are essential not just for case management but also for surveillance of disease trends. Such data may be used to justify implementing vector control or personal protection programmes, and to assess the impact of control interventions. When refugees or displaced people are settled in numerous camps or communities, consolidated microscopy and population data may be used as an indicator of which camps should be given priority for targeting interventions. The monitoring and quality control of field laboratories by a central reference laboratory is essential in ensuring an accurate diagnosis.

Table 5.10 **Minimum information required to investigate a suspected malaria outbreak**

Population
- Who is affected?
- Where are they from?
- How are they living?

Disease
- Number with acute febrile illness
- Number with confirmed uncomplicated malaria
- Number with microscopically confirmed severe malaria
- Number of malaria deaths
- Number of maternal deaths due to malaria
- Proportion of children with anaemia
- Proportion of pregnant women with anaemia
- Drug resistance; proportion of treatment failures

Management
- Number of health facilities (peripheral and referral)
- Available staff and expertise
- Access of population to the health facilities
- Availability of drugs and supplies
- Malaria policy and treatment guidelines

Monitoring malaria burden

Epidemiological information systems are essential in all malaria control programmes to assess the country's malaria situation, allow the forecasting of epidemics, define risk groups and monitor programme progress.

Further reading

Nájera JA. Malaria control among refugees and displaced populations. Geneva, World Health Organization, 1996 (document CTD/MAL/96.6).

Management of severe malaria – a practical handbook, 2nd ed. Geneva, World Health Organization, 2000.

The use of antimalarial drugs. Geneva, World Health Organization, 2001 (document WHO/CDS/RBM/2001.33).

Best practice and lessons learnt: implementing malaria control in complex emergencies in Africa 2000–2004. WHO/RBM Consultation, 15–17 November 2004, Geneva (document WHO/HTM/MAL/2005).

5.13 Measles

Basic facts

- Measles is a highly communicable viral infection spread via respiratory droplets from person to person.
- It is a severe disease caused by the *rubeola* virus, which damages epithelial surfaces and the immune system.
- Measles can increase susceptibility to other infectious agents such as pneumococcus, *Haemophilus influenzae* and *Staphylococcus aureus*.
- It can lead to or exacerbate vitamin A deficiency, thus increasing the risk of xerophthalmia, blindness and premature death.
- The most vulnerable are children between the ages of 9 months and 5 years in developing countries, but this depends on vaccination coverage rates.
- Deaths are mostly due to complications such as pneumonia, croup and diarrhoea and are frequently associated with malnutrition.

Natural history

- The incubation period is usually 10–12 days from exposure to onset of fever.
- Initial symptoms and signs are high fever, runny nose, coryza, cough, red eyes and Koplik spots (small white spots on the buccal mucosa).
- A characteristic erythematous (red) maculopapular (blotchy) rash appears on the third to seventh day, commencing behind the ears and on the hairline and then spreading to the rest of the body.
- The temperature subsides after 3–4 days and the rash fades after 5–6 days.
- Measles is highly infectious from the start of the prodromal period until approximately 4–5 days after the rash appears.
- Case-fatality rates are estimated at 3–5% in developing countries, but may be as high as 10–30% in displaced populations.

Complications

- Some 5–10% of patients develop complications.

- Complications occurring in the first week of the illness, such as croup, diarrhoea and pneumonia, are usually due to the effects of the measles virus and are rarely life-threatening.

- Later complications are usually due to secondary viral or bacterial infections. Post-measles pneumonia, diarrhoea and croup are the most common life-threatening complications (see Table 5.11).

Table 5.11   **Complications of measles**

Pneumonia	Usually severe, frequent bacterial superinfection
Diarrhoea	Caused either by the virus or by a secondary infection, e.g. *Shigella*
Malnutrition	Precipitated by anorexia, stomatitis, fever, vomiting, diarrhoea and other
Stomatitis	Compromises sucking and eating
Vitamin A deficiency	Keratoconjunctivitis; measles increases the need for vitamin A and often precipitates xerophthalmia and/or blindness due to scarring
Encephalitis	Acute measles encephalitis occurs in approximately 1 in 1000 infected children, typically during convalescence NB: the most common neurological manifestation of measles infection is febrile convulsions
Otitis media	This is a common complication of measles: the ear is painful and hearing is reduced
Croup	Laryngotracheobronchitis causing airway obstruction
Subacute sclerosing panencephalitis	Subacute sclerosing panencephalitis (SSPE) occurs in approximately 1 in 1 000 000 Onset is late, usually after 2–10 years

Case management

A history should be taken from the mother and the child should be examined for the signs and symptoms set out in Table 5.12.

Table 5.12   **Symptoms and signs indicating measles**

Symptoms	Signs
Ability to take feeds or fluids	Nutritional status
Cough and difficult breathing	Breathing rate, chest indrawing, stridor
Diarrhoea or blood in stools	Dehydration and fever
Sore mouth, eyes or ears	Mouth ulcers, sore and discharging ears and eyes, Bitot's spots[a] Level of consciousness

^a *Bitot's spots are superficial, foamy gray or white, irregularly shaped patches, which appear on the conjunctiva (or white) of the eyeball. They are due to severe vitamin A deficiency.*

Case management of uncomplicated measles: health centre

Most children will have uncomplicated measles and require supportive care as outpatients. Good supportive care can improve a child's outcome. Isolation of patients with measles is not indicated in emergency situations. All children with measles in these settings should have their nutritional status monitored and be enrolled in a selective feeding programme if necessary.

- The child should be nursed in a shaded and well ventilated area, as this is generally more comfortable for the child. Sunlight can be painful for the eyes and a cool environment can keep the temperature down.
- Control the fever by tepid sponging and administration of paracetamol.
- Keep the patient well hydrated; treat diarrhoea with oral rehydration salts.
- Observe the patient closely for complications.
- Give prophylaxis against xerophthalmia: vitamin A on days 1 and 2 (see Table 5.13).

Table 5.13 **Dosages of vitamin A in measles treatment regimens**

Age	Immediately on diagnosis	Following day
Infants < 6 months	50 000 IU	50 000 IU
Infants 6–11 months	100 000 IU	100 000 IU
Children > 11 months	200 000 IU	200 000 IU

- Maintain an adequate protein–calorie intake: inform mothers of the importance of frequent small meals.
- Continue breastfeeding.
- Provide supplementary feeding if available. The diet must be soft with a high calorie density, so that small portions go a long way. Protein, unless in the form of egg, is unlikely to be eaten (remember the child has a sore mouth and poor appetite).
- Do not admit patients to *general* feeding centres until after the infectious period.
- If there are large numbers of cases it may be necessary to set up a small unit for children with measles, as they and their mothers need a lot of supportive care.
- Use antimicrobials only when indicated.
- Undertake active case-finding during the epidemic, if practical (home visits).

Case management of complicated measles: health centre/hospital

- Control fever, provide nutritional support and ensure two doses of vitamin A have been given (as for uncomplicated measles).

- A third dose must be given after 2 weeks.

- Antimicrobials should not be given routinely.

- Indications for antimicrobial therapy are of two types: (*a*) documented complications such as pneumonia, otitis media and dysentery; and (*b*) children at significant risk of secondary bacterial infection (e.g. severe malnutrition, HIV infection or xerophthalmia). A broad-spectrum antimicrobial such as ampicillin or co-trimoxazole should be used.

- In case of cough and rapid breathing (40 breaths per minute or more if over 1 year of age; 50 breaths per minute if less than 1 year) give an antimicrobial such as ampicillin, amoxicillin or co-trimoxazole. If the child's condition does not improve after 24–48 hours, change the antimicrobial to an antistaphylococcal drug such as cloxacillin or chloramphenicol.

- If there are three or more loose or watery stools in 24 hours, assess for associated dehydration. If there is blood in the stool, the child has dysentery. The commonest cause of dysentery is *Shigella* spp. (see Section 5.2 for details of managing cases of shigellosis).

- The major eye problems associated with measles are measles conjunctivitis, or keratitis with ensuing corneal damage due to vitamin A deficiency. The mere observation of red and watery eyes without other complications does not justify specific treatment. Sticky eyes and pus in the eyes are due to secondary bacterial infection: clean the eye at least three times a day with cooled boiled water, using cotton wool or a clean cloth. Use tetracycline ointment three times a day for 7 days.

IMPORTANT. NEVER use steroid eye ointments.

Prevention and control measures

See Section 2.6.4.

IMPORTANT. While this section details the diagnosis and case management of measles, vaccination remains the most important strategy for measles control. Measles vaccination campaigns are one of the highest priorities in emergency situations.

Further reading

Conduite à tenir en cas d'épidémie de rougeole.[Management of a measles outbreak] Paris, Médecins Sans Frontières, 1996.

Treating measles in children. Geneva, World Health Organization, 1997 (document WHO/EPI/TRAM/97.02).

WHO-UNICEF joint statement on reducing measles mortality in emergencies (document WHO/V&B/04.03 or UNICEF/PD/Measles/02).

Measles Technical Working Group: Strategies for measles control and elimination. Report of a meeting. 11–12 May 2000. Genenva, World Health Organization 2001 (document WHO/V&B/01.37).

5.14 Meningococcal meningitis (epidemic)

Basic facts

- Meningococcal meningitis is an acute inflammation of the meninges, usually caused by bacteria.
- Large outbreaks of meningitis are mainly due to the meningococcus *Neisseria meningitidis* (serogroups A, C and, more recently, W135+A+C).
- *N. meningitidis* also causes meningococcal septicaemia, a severe disease with signs of acute fever, purpura and shock. It is less common but the case-fatality rate is high.
- *N. meningitidis*, *Streptococcus pneumoniae* and *Haemophilus influenzae* account for 80% of all cases of bacterial meningitis.
- Viral meningitis is rarely serious and may be caused by any of a number of viruses (such as coxsackie virus or enterovirus).
- Displaced populations are at increased risk of meningitis owing to over-crowding, poor hygiene and poor access to health care.
- Epidemics in refugee camps have mainly been due to *N. meningitidis* serogroup A.
- Endemic attack rates in sub-Saharan Africa range from under 10 to over 20 per 100 000 population.
- Epidemic attack rates in Africa can be as high as 1000 per 100 000 population.
- Some 80% of cases of meningococcal meningitis occur in those under 30 years of age.
- Without appropriate treatment, the case-fatality rate in meningococcal meningitis can be as high as 50%; with treatment this can be reduced to 5–15%.
- Vaccines are available against meningococcus A, C, Y and W135, and these are very effective in controlling epidemics. When used in rapid mass campaigns, vaccination can contain an outbreak within 2–3 weeks. The vaccine efficacy rate is 90% one week after injection for those over 2 years of age.

Clinical features

The clinical case definition is sudden onset of fever (> 38.0 °C axillary) and one of the following: neck stiffness, altered consciousness; other meningeal sign; or petechial or purpural rash.

In patients under 1 year of age, meningitis is suspected when fever is accompanied by a bulging fontanelle.

Diagnosis

Lumbar puncture is necessary to determine whether acute meningitis is bacterial, and to identify the meningococcus (and exclude other causative pathogens, such as pneumococcus and *H. influenzae*). Lumbar puncture should be done as soon as meningitis is suspected before starting antimicrobial treatment.

In bacterial meningitis, the cerebrospinal fluid is usually cloudy or purulent (but may be clear or bloody). The basic laboratory examination consists of a white cell count (WCC), protein concentration and Gram stain.

Several new rapid diagnostic tests are available that can be useful in confirming meningococcal meningitis including serotypes A, C, Y, and W135 of *Neisseria meningitidis*.

Meningococcal meningitis if:

WCC > 1000 cells/mm³ (<3 in normal CSF) with >60% polymorphs.

Protein concentration > 0.80 g/l (< 0.60 g/l in normal CSF).

Gram stain: Gram-negative diplococci (intra- or extracellular) in 80% of cases not previously treated.

Differential diagnosis

A lumbar puncture should be performed and the cerebrospinal fluid examined to differentiate viral from bacterial meningitis (see Annex 8 for guidelines on collection of CSF specimens).

Thick and thin smears should be made to differentiate meningococcal meningitis from cerebral malaria in malaria-endemic areas.

Case management

- Bacterial meningitis, particularly meningococcal meningitis, is potentially fatal and is a medical emergency.
- Viral meningitis is rarely serious and requires supportive care, but a lumbar puncture is necessary to differentiate it from bacterial meningitis.
- All suspected meningitis patients should be admitted to hospital or a health centre for diagnosis and case management.
- Antimicrobial treatment should be started immediately after taking a lumbar puncture without waiting for the results.
- Treatment with antimicrobials should not be delayed if lumbar puncture cannot be performed.

- Intravenous administration of benzylpenicillin, ampicillin, ceftriaxone or cefotaxime is recommended for bacterial meningitis.
- In patients for whom the intramuscular or intravenous route is not possible, oral administration is acceptable but higher doses are necessary.
- During large epidemics among refugees or displaced populations, a single-dose regimen of oily chloramphenicol intramuscularly can be used if resources or circumstances do not permit the administration of a full course of standard treatment.

Table 5.14 **Initial empirical antimicrobial therapy for presumed bacterial meningitis**

Age group	Probable pathogens	Antimicrobial therapy	
		First choice	Alternative
Epidemic situations			
All age groups	*N. meningitidis*	Benzylpenicillin *or* oily chloramphenicol	Ampicillin *or* ceftriaxone *or* cefotaxime *or* co-trimoxazole
Non-epidemic situations			
Adults and children > 5 years	*N. meningitidis* *S. pneumoniae*	Benzylpenicillin *or* oily chloramphenicol	Ampicillin *or* ceftriaxone *or* cefotaxime *or* co-trimoxazole
Children 1 month to 5 years	*H. influenzae* *S. pneumoniae* *N. meningitidis*	Ampicilin *or* amoxycilin *or* chloramphenicol	Ceftriaxone *or* cefotaxime
Neonates	Gram-negative bacteria Group B streptococci *Listeria* spp.	Ampicillin *and* gentamicin	Ceftriaxone *or* cefotaxime *or* chloramphenicol

- In meningococcal septicaemia with purpura and shock, shock should be treated by restoring blood volume.
- Chemoprophylaxis of contacts is not recommended in emergency situations.
- Supportive therapy should be given to maintain hydration and adequate nutrition.
- Convulsions should be treated with diazepam, intravenously or rectally.
- The patient should be nursed in a shaded and well-ventilated area. The unconscious or semiconscious patient should be nursed on his/her side; turning every 2–3 hours can prevent pressure sores.

Table 5.15   **Antimicrobials to treat bacterial meningitis**

Agent	Route	Daily dose, adults	Daily dose, children	Duration (days)
Benzylpenicillin	IV	3–4 MU four–six times	400 000 U/kg	> 4
Ampicillin/ amoxicillin	IV	2–3 g twice	250 mg/kg	> 4
Amoxicillin	Oral	2–3 g twice	250 mg/kg	> 4
Chloramphenicol	IV	1 g twice–three times	100 mg/kg	> 4
Chloramphenicol (oily)	IM	3 g single dose	100 mg/kg	1–2
Cefotaxime	IV	2 g twice	250 mg/kg	> 4
Ceftriaxone	IV	1–2 g once–twice	50–80 mg/kg	> 4
Ceftriaxone	IM	1–2 g single dose	50–80 mg/kg	1–2
Co-trimoxazole	IV/IM	2 g SMZ twice [a]	100 mg/kg	> 4
Co-trimoxazole	Oral	2 g SMZ twice [a]	100 mg/kg	> 4
Sulfadiazine	IV	1 g six times	200 mg/kg	> 4

[a] *SMZ = sulfamethoxazole*

Prevention and control measures

See Section 4.2.2 for detecting an outbreak of meningococcal meningitis (alert and epidemic thresholds). See Section 2.6.5 for implementing a mass vaccination campaign.

Further reading

Conduite à tenir en cas d'épidémie de méningite à méningocoque [Management of a meningococcal meningitis outbreak]. Paris, Médecins Sans Frontières, 1996.

Control of epidemic meningococcal diseases: WHO practical guidelines, 2nd ed. Geneva, World Health Organization, 1998 (document WHO/EMC/BAC/98.3).

Detecting meningococcal meningitis epidemics in highly-endemic African countries: WHO recommendation. *Weekly Epidemiological Record*, 2000, **38**:306–309.

Emergence of W135 meningococcal disease. Report of a WHO Consultation, Geneva, 17–18 September 2001. Geneva, World Health Organization, 2001 (document WHO/CDS/CSR/GAR/2002.1).

Laboratory methods for the diagnosis of meningitis caused by Neisseria meningitidis, Streptococcus pneumoniae, and Haemophilus influenzae. Geneva, World Health Organization, 1999 (document WHO/CDS/CSR/EDC/99.7).

5.15 Relapsing fever (louse-borne)

Basic facts

- Relapsing fever is a severe febrile disease, usually lasting 2–3 weeks.
- Epidemic relapsing fever is caused by *Borrelia recurrentis*, a bacterium that is transmitted by body lice.
- Although it is present sporadically in almost all continents (except Oceania), relapsing fever is endemic in Sudan and in the highlands of Ethiopia.
- Periods of fever usually last 4–6 days and alternate with afebrile periods.
- Each febrile period is terminated by a crisis.
- The incubation period is about a week.
- Up to 20% of untreated patients die.

Diagnosis

- In endemic areas, under conditions of overcrowding and very poor sanitation, a health worker should suspect relapsing fever in a patient with high fever and two of the following four symptoms:
  - severe joint pain,
  - chills,
  - jaundice,
  - nose or other bleeding,

  or in a patient with high fever who is responding poorly to antimalarial drugs.
- In areas where there have been no cases for a number of months, it is advisable to confirm the initial cases in the laboratory by microscopy.
- The diagnosis of relapsing fever can be confirmed by taking blood from patients suspected of having the disease while they have acute high fever, and sending to a laboratory where testing can be carried out. Typical *Borrelia* spirochaetes can be seen directly through blood-smear microscopy.
- The seams of clothing should be examined for lice and their eggs. Very often the children of the household will easily be able to identify lice in the clothing if present. Blankets and any changes of clothing should be checked.

Case management

- Effective treatment is available, comprising a single dose of a common antimicrobial (e.g. erythromycin, tetracycline or doxycycline), as follows:
  - doxycycline: single dose of 100 mg in adults,
  - tetracycline: single dose of 500 mg in adults,
  - erythromycin: single dose of 500 mg in adults and children over 5 years,
  - erythromycin: single dose of 250 mg in children up to 5 years.

IMPORTANT. Doxycycline and tetracycline must **not** be given to pregnant women.

Prevention and control measures
- Detect and treat all those suspected of having relapsing fever and their close contacts.
- Carry out a population-based delousing programme in affected areas.
- Promote improved personal hygiene.
- Prevent further outbreaks through community prevention programmes.
- Control body louse infestation (see Sections 2.4.1 and 5.21).

5.16 Scabies

Basic facts
- Scabies is a parasitic disease of the skin caused by the mite *Sarcoptes scabiei*.
- It is transmitted by direct skin-to-skin contact or sexual contact.
- Transfer from bedclothes can occur only if clothing has been contaminated by an infested person immediately beforehand.
- The infestation presents as papules, vesicles or burrows containing the mites and their eggs.
- Lesions are most common around finger webs, wrists and elbows and the abdomen.
- The head, neck, palms and soles may be affected in infants.
- The disease has widespread distribution.
- The largest epidemics have occurred in conditions of poor sanitation and overcrowding following displacement.
- Scabies is endemic in most developing countries.

Clinical features
- In people without previous exposure, the incubation period is 2–6 weeks before the onset of itching.
- In previously infested people, symptoms occur 1–4 days after re-exposure.
- Intense itching occurs especially at night.
- Scratching can be severe in children, and result in secondary bacterial infection of the papules.
- Infestation can be severe and debilitating in malnourished people.

Diagnosis

- Clinical diagnosis is made by the identification of characteristic lesions.
- Mites recovered from burrows can be identified microscopically.

Case management

- Treatment of the whole group is necessary, as some members maybe asymptomatic.
- Formulations of insecticides (below) can be applied as creams, lotions or aqueous emulsions for use against scabies. The formulation must be applied to all parts of the body below the neck, not only to the places where itching is felt. It should not be washed off until the next day. Treated persons can dress after the application has been allowed to dry for about 15 minutes.
- Malathion (1%) aqueous emulsion or permethrin (5%) cream should be applied to the body below the neck and left for 24 hours before washing.
- Gamma benzene hexachloride cream (1%) may also be used.
- Benzyl benzoate (25%) emulsion may be used but may require repeated applications. Half- and quarter-strength solutions should be used for children aged 8–12 and 4–7 years, respectively.
- Benzyl benzoate is irritating and should be avoided in malnourished children where possible. Benzyl benzoate should also be avoided if possible if the patient has open lesions due to scratching.
- Clothing and bedclothes should be washed if possible.
- Ivermectin, used for filariasis and onchocerciasis, is also effective in treating scabies infections in a single oral dose of 100–200 mg/kg body weight. It can be particularly useful in outbreaks, in HIV-infected individuals and in crusted scabies.

5.17 Sexually transmitted infections

Basic facts

The four main syndromes of sexually transmitted infections (STIs) are:

- urethral discharge,
- vaginal discharge,
- genital ulcer disease,
- lower abdominal pain.

Syndromic management of STIs is particularly relevant in resource-poor settings and in emergency situations, where laboratory back-up of clinical diagnosis is seldom available. A number of algorithms (flow charts) have been proposed for the four syndromes listed above. Their performance is better for urethral discharge and genital ulcer disease. Current algorithms for vaginal discharge are not highly effective in detecting gonorrhoea and chlamydial infection in women, or in discriminating between vaginal infections and vaginal plus cervical infections. WHO algorithms for urethral discharge, genital ulcers and vaginal discharge are described in Annex 13.

Prevention of STIs is an important control measure and consists of:

- early diagnosis and treatment of women and men and management of partners;
- health education: safe sexual behaviour messages in health education activities and promotion of appropriate health-care-seeking behaviour;
- condom distribution.

Specific diagnosis and case management

Genital ulcer

Genital ulcers may be due to syphilis, chancroid, granuloma inguinale or herpes simplex. Clinical differential diagnosis of genital ulcers is inaccurate, particularly in settings where several etiologies are common. Clinical manifestations may be further altered in the presence of HIV infection.

The patient should be examined to confirm the presence of genital ulceration. Treatment appropriate to local etiologies and antimicrobial sensitivity patterns should be given. For example, in areas where more than one cause is known to be present, patients with genital ulcers should be treated for all relevant conditions at the time of their initial presentation to ensure adequate therapy in case of loss to follow-up.

Laboratory-assisted differential diagnosis is rarely helpful at the initial visit, and mixed infections are common. For instance, in areas of high syphilis incidence, a reactive serological test may reflect a previous infection and give a misleading picture of the patient's present condition.

Recommended regimens:
- treatment for syphilis

plus
- treatment for chancroid **or** treatment for granuloma inguinale

---

Genital ulcer and HIV infection

In HIV-infected patients, prolonged courses of treatment may be necessary for chancroid. Moreover, where HIV infection is prevalent, a significant proportion of patients with genital ulcer may also carry herpes simplex virus. Herpetic ulcers may be atypical and persist for long periods in HIV-infected patients.

Patients with genital ulcers should be followed up weekly until the ulceration shows signs of healing.

Urethral discharge

Male patients with urethral discharge and/or dysuria should be examine for evidence of discharge.

If microscopy is available, a urethral specimen should be taken and a urethral smear stained with Gram stain. A count of more than 5 polymorphonuclear leukocytes per field ($\times$ 1000) confirms a diagnosis of urethritis.

The major pathogens causing urethral discharge are *Neisseria gonorrhoeae* and *Chlamydia trachomatis*. Unless a diagnosis of gonorrhoea can be definitively excluded by laboratory tests, the treatment of the patient with urethral discharge should provide adequate coverage of these two organisms.

Recommended regimens:
- treat as for uncomplicated gonorrhoea

plus
- doxycycline, 100 mg orally, twice daily for 7 days
  or tetracycline, 500 mg orally, four times daily for 7 days

Note: Tetracyclines are contraindicated in pregnancy.

Alternative regimen where single-dose therapy for gonorrhoea is not available:
- trimethoprim (80 mg) + sulfamethoxazole (400 mg), 10 tablets orally, daily for 3 days

plus
- doxycycline, 100 mg orally, twice daily for 7 days
  or tetracycline, 500 mg orally, four times daily for 7 days

Note: This regimen should be used only in areas where trimethoprim–sulfamethoxazole has been shown to be effective against uncomplicated gonorrhoea.

Alternative if tetracyclines are contraindicated or not tolerated:
- treat as for uncomplicated gonorrhoea

plus
- erythromycin, 500 mg orally, four times daily for 7 days

As follow-up, patients should be advised to return if symptoms persist 7 days after the start of therapy.

Vaginal discharge

Vaginal discharge is most commonly caused by vaginitis, but may also be the result of cervicitis. Vaginitis may be caused by *Trichomonas vaginalis*, *Candida albicans* and a combination of *Gardnerella* spp. and anaerobic bacterial infection (bacterial vaginosis).

Cervicitis may be due to *N. gonorrhoeae* or *Chlamydia trachomatis* infection. Management is more important than that of vaginitis, from a public health point of view, as cervicitis may have serious sequelae. However, clinical differentiation between the two conditions is difficult and ideally requires speculum examination by a skilled physician.

Cervicitis

Recommended regimens:
- treat as for uncomplicated gonorrhoea

plus
- doxycycline, 100 mg orally, twice daily for 7 days
  or tetracycline, 500 mg orally, four times daily for 7 days

Note: Tetracyclines are contraindicated in pregnancy.

Alternative if tetracyclines are contraindicated or not tolerated:
- treat as for uncomplicated gonorrhoea

plus
- erythromycin, 500 mg orally, four times daily for 7 days

Alternative regimen where single-dose therapy for gonorrhoea is not available:
- trimethoprim (80 mg) + sulfamethoxazole (400 mg), 10 tablets orally, daily for 3 days

plus
- doxycycline, 100 mg orally, twice daily for 7 days
  or tetracycline, 500 mg orally, four times daily for 7 days

Note. This regimen should be used only in areas where trimethoprim–sulfamethoxazole has been shown to be effective against uncomplicated gonorrhoea.

Vaginitis

Recommended regimens:

- treat with metronidazole, 2 g orally as a single dose
  or metronidazole, 400–500 mg orally, twice daily for 7 days

plus

- nystatin, 100 000 IU intravaginally, once daily for 14 days
  or miconazole or clotrimazole, 200 mg intravaginally, once daily for 3 days
  or clotrimazole, 500 mg intravaginally, as a single dose

Note: Patients taking metronidazole should be cautioned to avoid alcohol.

Lower abdominal pain

All sexually active women presenting with lower abdominal pain should be carefully evaluated for the presence of salpingitis and/or endometritis–pelvic inflammatory disease (PID). In addition, routine bimanual and abdominal examinations should be carried out on all women with a presumptive STI, since some women with PID or endometritis will not complain of lower abdominal pain. Women with endometritis may present with complaints of vaginal discharge and/or bleeding and/or uterine tenderness on pelvic examination. Symptoms suggestive of PID include abdominal pain, dyspareunia, vaginal discharge, menometrorrhagia, dysuria, pain associated with menses, fever, and sometimes nausea and vomiting.

PID is generally caused by *N. gonorrhoeae*, *C. trachomatis* and anaerobic bacteria (*Bacteroides* spp. and Gram-positive cocci). It is difficult to diagnose because clinical manifestations are varied. PID becomes highly probable when one or more of the above symptoms are seen in a woman with adnexal tenderness, evidence of lower genital tract infection and cervical motion tenderness. Enlargement or induration of one or both fallopian tubes, tender pelvic mass, and direct or rebound tenderness may also be present. The patient's temperature may be elevated but is normal in many cases. In general, clinicians should err on the side of over-diagnosing and treating milder cases.

Patients with acute PID should be admitted to hospital if:

- the diagnosis is uncertain,
- surgical emergencies such as appendicitis and ectopic pregnancy need to be excluded,
- a pelvic abscess is suspected,
- severe illness precludes management on an outpatient basis,
- the patient is pregnant,
- the patient is unable to follow or tolerate an outpatient regimen,
- the patient has failed to respond to outpatient therapy,
- clinical follow-up 72 hours after the start of antimicrobial treatment cannot be guaranteed.

See recommended regimens for lower abdominal pain related to sexually transmitted diseases below.

Further reading

Guidelines for the management of sexually transmitted infections. Geneva, World Health Organization, 2001 (document WHO/HIV_AIDS/2001.01).

Dallabetta GA, Laga M, Lamptey PR. *Control of sexually transmitted diseases: a handbook for the design and management of programs*. Arlington, VA, AIDSCAP Project, Family Health International, 1997.

Lower abdominal pain

INPATIENT THERAPY: recommended syndromic treatment (3 alternative regimens)

1. ceftriaxone, 250 mg intramuscularly, once daily
   plus doxycycline, 100 mg orally or intravenously, twice daily
   or tetracycline, 500 mg orally, 4 times daily

2. clindamycin, 900 mg intravenously, every 8 hours
   plus gentamicin, 1.5 mg/kg intravenously every 8 hours

3. ciprofloxacin, 500 mg orally, twice daily, or spectinomycin 1 g intramuscularly, 4 times daily
   plus metronidazole, 400–500 mg orally or intravenously, twice daily
   or chloramphenicol, 500 mg orally or intravenously, 4 times daily

Note: For all three regimens, continue treatment for at least 2 days after the patient has improved and follow with:

• doxycycline, 100 mg orally, twice daily for 14 days
  or tetracycline, 500 mg orally, four times daily for 14 days

Note: Patients taking metronidazole should be cautioned to avoid alcohol. Tetracyclines are contraindicated in pregnancy.

OUTPATIENT THERAPY: recommended syndromic treatment

• single-dose therapy for uncomplicated gonorrhoea

plus

• doxycycline, 100 mg orally, twice daily for 14 days
  or tetracycline, 500 mg orally, four times daily for 14 days

plus

• metronidazole, 400–500 mg orally, twice daily for 14 days

Note: Patients taking metronidazole should be cautioned to avoid alcohol. Tetracyclines are contraindicated in pregnancy.

Outpatients with PID should be followed up at 72 hours and admitted if their condition has not improved.

OUTPATIENT THERAPY: alternative syndromic treatment where single-dose therapy for gonorrhoea is not available:

- trimethoprim (80 mg) + sulfamethoxazole (400 mg), 10 tablets orally once daily for 3 days and then 2 tablets orally twice daily for 10 days

plus

- doxycycline 100 mg orally, twice daily
  or tetracycline 500 mg orally, 4 times daily for 14 days

plus

- metronidazole 400–500 mg orally, twice daily for 14 days

Note: This regimen should be used only in areas where trimethoprim–sulfamethoxazole has been shown to be effective in the treatment of uncomplicated gonorrhoea. Patients taking metronidazole should be cautioned to avoid alcohol. Tetracyclines are contraindicated in pregnancy.

Outpatients with PID should be followed up at 72 hours and admitted if their condition has not improved.

5.18 Trypanosomiasis, African (African sleeping sickness)[6]

Basic facts

- African trypanosomiasis is found uniquely in sub-Saharan Africa. In epidemic situations, as in the Democratic Republic of the Congo, the prevalence of the disease can be as high as 70% in some areas.

- An important feature of African trypanosomiasis is its focal nature. It tends to occur in circumscribed zones. Observed prevalence ratios vary greatly from one geographical area to another, and even between one village and another within the same area.

- War and displacement are not directly involved in the spread of the disease, but they play a major role in causing the breakdown of surveillance, case-detection and treatment.

- The causal agents are:

  - *Trypanosoma brucei gambiense* (tropical forest, central and west Africa);

  - *T. b. rhodesiense* (savannah, east and southern Africa).

- Endemic countries can be classified into four major levels of endemicity depending on their level of disease prevalence (see map below. Even within each country the spacial distribution is highly heterogeneous and occurs in foci and micro-foci.

---

[6] American trypanosomiasis (Chagas disease) is unlikely to be a problem in emergencies and will not be discussed here.

Human African Trypanosomiasis

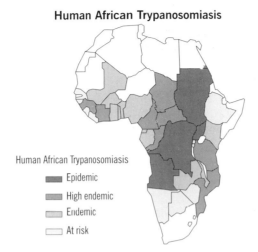

Human African Trypanosomiasis
- ▬ Epidemic
- ▬ High endemic
- ▬ Endemic
- ☐ At risk

- Humans are the major reservoir in the *T. b. gambiense* form; wild ruminants and domestic cattle are the major reservoir for *T. b. rhodesiense*. Outbreaks occur when human–fly contact is intensified or through movements of hosts or infected flies.

- Infection occurs after an infected tsetse fly (*Glossina* spp.) bites the victim and transmits the trypanosome. The parasite then multiplies in the blood and lymph glands and, after a variable delay, crosses the blood–brain barrier and provokes major, often irreversible, neurological disorders that lead to death. The incubation period is short for *T. b. rhodesiense* (3 days to a few weeks); it can be years for *T. b. gambiense*.

Clinical features

In the early stages, a painful chancre (rare in *T. b. gambiense* infection), which originates as a papule and evolves into a nodule, may be found at the primary site of a tsetse fly bite. There may be fever, intense headache, insomnia, painless lymphadenopathy, anaemia, local oedema and rash. In the later stage there is cachexia, sleep disturbance and signs of central nervous system impairment. The disease may run a protracted course of several years in the case of *T. b. gambiense*. In the case of *T. b. rhodesiense*, the disease has a rapid and acute evolution. Both diseases are always fatal in the absence of treatment.

Diagnosis

- Presumptive: serological: card agglutination trypanosomiasis test (CATT): for *T. b. gambiense* only or immunofluorescent assay for *T. b. rhodesiense* mainly and possibly for *T. b. gambiense*.

- Confirmative: parasitological: detection (microscopy) of trypanosomes in blood, lymph node aspirates or CSF.

Case management

Early screening and diagnosis are essential, as treatment is easier in the first stage of the disease (fewer injections required, no psychiatric disorders), carries a lower risk and can be administered on an outpatient basis. Diagnosis and treatment require trained personnel, and self-treatment is not possible. Most available drugs are old, difficult to administer where resources are limited, and by no means always successful.

T. b. gambiense

Recommended regimens

- **First stage of the disease (without cerebrospinal fluid involvement)**
  Pentamidine (4 mg/kg body weight per day) intramuscularly for 7 consecutive days on an outpatient basis.

- **Second stage (with cerebrospinal fluid involvement)**
  Melarsoprol – Hospitalization with 3 series of daily injections administered with a rest period of 8 to 10 days between each series. A series consists of one injection of 3.6 mg/kg/daily melarsoprol intravenously for 3 consecutive days.

  In case of melarsoprol treatment failure, use *eflornithine* 400 mg/kg per day administered in four daily slow infusions (lasting approximately 2 hours). Infusions are given every 6 hours, which represents a dose of 100 mg/kg per infusion.

T. b. rhodesiense

Recommended regimens

- **First stage of the disease (without cerebrospinal fluid involvement)**
  Suramin – The recommended dosage is 20 mg/kg per day with a maximum dose of 1 g per injection. The drug is administered intravenously at the rate of one injection per week. The treatment course is 5 weeks for a total of 5 injections.

- **Second stage of the disease (with cerebrospinal fluid involvement)**
  Melarsoprol – Hospitalization with 3 series of daily injections administered with a rest period of 8 – 10 days between each series. A series consists of one injection of 3.6 mg/kg per day melarsoprol intravenously for 3 consecutive days.

Note: Melarsoprol causes reactive encephalopathy in 5–10% of patients, with fatal outcome in about half the cases. The treatment has a 10–30% rate of treatment failure, probably due to pharmacological resistance.

Increasing rates of *resistance to melarsoprol* (as high as 25%) have been reported from various African countries, such as Sudan and Uganda, leading to greater use of *eflornithine*.

Procurement of equipment and drugs

Since 2001, a public-private partnership agreement signed by WHO has made all these drugs widely available. The drugs are donated to WHO. Requests for supplies are made to WHO by governments of disease-endemic countries and organizations working in associations with these governments. Stock control and delivery of the drugs are undertaken by Médecins Sans Frontières in accordance with WHO guidelines. All the drugs are provided free of charge: recipient countries pay only for transport costs and customs charges.

Prevention

- Human reservoirs should be contained through periodic population screening and chemotherapy.
- Tsetse fly control programmes should be conducted, using traps and screens (may be impregnated with insecticide).
- Public education should be undertaken on personal protection against the bites of the tsetse fly.
- Donation of blood by those who live or have stayed in endemic areas should be prohibited.

Control measures in epidemic situations

Control measures comprise surveys to identify affected areas; early identification of infection in the community, followed by treatment; and urgent implementation of tsetse fly control measures.

Drug resistance monitoring

Melarsoprol treatment failure can be as high as 30% in some areas. A melarsoprol resistance surveillance network has been established by WHO.

Further reading

WHO report on global surveillance of epidemic-prone infectious diseases: African trypanosomiasis. Geneva, WHO, 2000 (WHO/CDS/CSR/ISR/2000.1).

Human trypanosomiasis: a guide for drug supply. Geneva, World Health Organization, 2001 (document WHO/CDS/CSR/EPH/2001.3).

Programme against African trypanosomiasis (PAAT), 2004. ISSN 1812:2442.

5.19 Tuberculosis

Basic facts

- Tuberculosis (TB) is a disease most commonly affecting the lungs, but also other organs.
- It is caused by the bacterium *Mycobacterium tuberculosis*. The *M. tuberculosis* complex includes *M. tuberculosis* and *M. africanum*, primarily from humans, and *M. bovis*, primarily from cattle.

- *M. tuberculosis* and *M. africanum* are transmitted by exposure to the bacilli in airborne droplet nuclei produced by people with pulmonary or laryngeal tuberculosis during expiratory efforts, such as coughing and sneezing.
- Bovine TB results from exposure to tuberculous cattle, usually by ingestion of unpasteurized milk or dairy products, and sometimes by airborne spread to farmers and animal handlers.
- The incubation period is about 2–10 weeks; latent infections may persist throughout a person's life.
- In the acute phase of an emergency, when mortality rates are high owing to acute respiratory infections, malnutrition, diarrhoeal diseases and malaria (where prevalent), TB control is not a priority. A TB control programme should not be implemented until crude mortality rates are below 1 per 10 000 population per day. It is crucial that there is some stability in the population, as all patients commencing TB treatment must complete the full 6- or 8-month treatment course. If there are high rates of treatment defaulters, there is a high risk of development of multidrug-resistant TB.
- Nevertheless, TB is a particularly important disease in long-term emergencies where refugees or internally displaced persons are in camps or overcrowded communities for long periods. In these conditions, people are at particularly high risk of developing TB owing to overcrowding, malnutrition and high HIV seroprevalence. In Kenya in 1993, the incidence of new infectious TB patients in camps was four times the rate in the local population. In two camps in Sudan in 1990, over one-third of all adult deaths were due to TB.

Diagnosis

The most important symptoms of TB are:

- productive cough of long duration (> 3 weeks),
- haemoptysis,
- significant weight loss.

TB patients may also have fever, night sweats, breathlessness, chest pain and loss of appetite.

The full case definitions for TB are given in Annex 5.

Patients with suspected TB should have three sputum samples examined by light microscopy for acid-fast bacilli, using the Ziehl-Neelsen stain.

Criteria for establishing a TB control programme in emergency situations

DOTS is the TB control strategy recommended by WHO. It is important that the TB programme implements the DOTS strategy and, where possible, coordinates this with the national TB programme of the host country. The same treatment protocols should be used, and data on case-finding and treatment outcome should be reported to the relevant district TB coordinator of the national TB programme. Implementation of a DOTS programme requires that the following criteria are met:

- case detection through sputum-smear microscopy; this implies the existence of a laboratory system capable of undertaking sputum-smear microscopy to an acceptable standard;
- standardized short-course chemotherapy available to at least all smear-positive patients under direct observation of treatment, at least during the initial phase of treatment;
- a secure and regular supply of appropriate anti-TB drugs;
- a monitoring system for programme supervision and evaluation;
- political willingness on the part of the relevant government(s) authorities to implement the programme.

The following criteria are essential before a TB programme is implemented:

- surveillance data indicate that TB is an important health problem;
- the acute emergency phase is over;
- the basic needs of water, adequate food, shelter and sanitation are met;
- essential clinical services and drugs are available;
- security in and stability of the affected population is envisaged for at least 6 months;
- sufficient funding is available to support the programme for at least 12 months;
- laboratory services for sputum-smear microscopy are available.

Once the decision to implement a DOTS programme is made, the following information should be collected:

- available funding and duration of support;
- annual TB incidence in the country of origin;
- TB control policies in the country of origin and the host country;
- expertise among the national TB programme or nongovernmental organizations in implementing TB control programmes.

Drug procurement, establishment of laboratory services and training may take up to 3 months, so the decision to implement a TB control programme should be made as soon as possible after the acute emergency phase is over.

The key steps in setting up a TB control programme using the DOTS strategy are:

- lead agency identified, e.g. national TB programme, nongovernmental organization;

- funding identified;
- work plan, resource needs and budget prepared;
- TB coordinator(s) (if possible 1 per 50 000 population) appointed;
- agreement with national TB programme of host country on:
  - integration of refugee/internally displaced person TB control programme with national TB programme,
  - drug regimens to be used,
  - coverage of the local population by the TB control programme,
  - referral of seriously ill patients to local hospitals,
  - laboratories suitable for quality control of smear examination,
  - procurement of drug stocks and reagents,
  - procedures for follow-up of cases in the repatriation phase,
  - programme evaluation;
- staff needs assessed, job descriptions developed and staff recruited;
- secure storage facilities identified;
- production of local TB control protocol;
- reporting system established.

Case management

The priority is the diagnosis and treatment of smear-positive infectious cases of TB. To ensure the appropriate treatment and cure of TB patients, strict implementation of the DOTS strategy is important.

There are primarily three types of regimen:

- category 1 for new smear-positive (infectious) pulmonary cases,
- category 2 for re-treatment cases,
- category 3 for smear-negative pulmonary or extra-pulmonary cases.

The chemotherapeutic regimens are based on standardized combinations of five essential drugs: rifampicin (R), isoniazid (H), pyrazinamide (P), ethambutol (E) and streptomycin (S).

Each of the standardized chemotherapeutic regimens consist of two phases:

- the initial (intensive) phase: 2–3 months, with 3–5 drugs given daily under direct observation;
- the continuation phase: 4–6 months, with 2–3 drugs given three times a week under direct observation, or in some cases (e.g. during repatriation of refugees) two drugs for 6 months given daily unsupervised, but in fixed-dose combination form.

All doses of rifampicin-containing regimens should be observed by staff. Actual swallowing of medication should be supervised.

Multidrug-resistant TB

- MDR-TB is a specific form of drug-resistant TB due to a bacillus resistant to at least isoniazid and rifampicin, the two most powerful anti-TB drugs.
- DOTS-Plus is designed to cure MDR-TB using second-line anti-TB drugs.
- DOTS-Plus is needed in areas where MDR-TB has emerged due to previous inadequate TB control programmes.
- DOTS-Plus pilot projects are **recommended only in settings where the DOTS strategy is fully in place to protect against the creation of further drug resistance.**
- It is vital that WHO is consulted before DOTS-Plus pilot projects are launched in order to minimize the risk of creating drug resistance to second-line anti-TB drugs.

Further reading

Harries AD, Maher D. *TB/HIV: a clinical manual*. Geneva, World Health Organization, 1996 (document WHO/TB/96.200).

Treatment of tuberculosis: guidelines for national programmes, 2nd ed. Geneva, World Health Organization, 1997 (document WHO/TB/97.220).

Tuberculosis control in refugee situations: an inter-agency field manual. Geneva, World Health Organization, 1997 (document WHO/TB/97.221).

5.20 Typhoid fever

Basic facts

- Typhoid fever is caused by *Salmonella* Typhi, a Gram-negative bacterium. A very similar but often less severe disease is caused by the *Salmonella* serotype Paratyphi A. In most countries in which these diseases have been studied, the ratio of disease caused by *S.* Typhi to that caused by *S.* Paratyphi is about 10:1.
- Typhoid fever remains a global health problem. It is difficult to estimate the real burden of typhoid fever in the world because the clinical picture is confused with many other febrile infections because of the lack of appropriate laboratory resources in most areas in developing countries. Many cases remain under-diagnosed. In both endemic areas and in large outbreaks, most cases of typhoid fever are seen in those aged 3–19 years.
- Humans are the only natural host and reservoir. The infection is transmitted by ingestion of faecally contaminated food or water. The highest incidence occurs where water supplies serving a large population are faecally contaminated.
- The incubation period is usually 8–14 days, but may extend from 3 days up to 2 months.

- Some 2–5% of infected people become chronic carriers who harbour *S.* Typhi in the gall bladder. Chronic carriers are greatly involved in the spread of the disease.
- Patients infected with HIV are at a significantly increased risk of severe disease due to *S.* Typhi and *S.* Paratyphi.

Clinical features

The clinical presentation of typhoid fever varies from a mild illness with low-grade fever, malaise and dry cough to a severe clinical picture with abdominal discomfort, altered mental status and multiple complications.

Clinical diagnosis is difficult. In the absence of laboratory confirmation, any case of fever of at least 38 °C for 3 or more days is considered suspect if the epidemiological context is conducive.

Depending on the clinical setting and quality of available medical care, some 5–10% of typhoid patients may develop serious complications, the most frequent being intestinal haemorrhage or peritonitis due to intestinal perforation.

Clinical case definitions are given in Table 5.16.

Table 5.16   **Clinical case definitions**

Confirmed case of typhoid fever	A patient with fever (38 °C or more) lasting 3 or more days, with laboratory-confirmed *S.* Typhi organisms (blood, bone marrow, bowel fluid)
Probable case of typhoid fever	A patient with fever (38 °C or more) lasting 3 or more days, with a positive serodiagnosis or antigen detection test but no *S.* Typhi isolation
Chronic carrier	An individual excreting *S.* Typhi in the stool or urine for longer than one year after the onset of acute typhoid fever; short-term carriers also exist, but their epidemiological role is not as important as that of chronic carriers

Diagnosis

✔ The definitive diagnosis of typhoid fever depends on the isolation of *S.* Typhi organisms from the blood or bone marrow or bowed fluid. Blood culture bottles should be transported to the referral laboratory at ambient temperature.

✔ The classical Widal test measuring agglutinating antibody titres against *S.* Typhi in serum has only moderate sensitivity and specificity. It can be negative in up to 30% of culture-proven cases of typhoid fever and can be falsely positive in many circumstances. Newer diagnostic tests based on detection of serum antibodies highly specific to *S.* Typhi are currently being developed and some have already been marketed. They are rapid, very accurate and easy to perform. Although they have not yet been evaluated extensively in the field, they are likely to become standard point-of-care tests for the diagnosis of typhoid fever, particularly in emergencies where access to blood culture facilities is compromised.

Case management

- More than 90% of patients can be managed at home with oral antimicrobial, minimal nursing care, and close medical follow-up for complications or failure to respond to therapy. However, the emergence of multidrug-resistant strains in many parts of the world has reduced the choice of effective anti-microbial available in many areas. When feasible, antimicrobial susceptibility testing is crucial as a guide to clinical management.

- The available evidence suggests that the fluoroquinolones[7] are the optimal choice for the treatment of typhoid fever at all ages. However, in areas of the world where the bacterium is still fully sensitive to traditional first-line drugs (chloramphenicol, ampicillin, amoxicillin or trimethoprim–sulfamethoxazole) and fluoroquinolones are not available or affordable, these drugs do remain appropriate for the treatment of typhoid fever. Chloramphenicol, despite the risk of agranulocytosis (1 per 10 000 patients), is still widely prescribed in developing countries to treat typhoid fever. S. Typhi strains from many areas of the world, such as Indonesia and most countries in Africa, remain sensitive to this drug.

- Supportive measures are important in the management of typhoid fever, such as oral or intravenous hydration, antipyretics, and appropriate nutrition and blood transfusions, if indicated.

- Typhoid fever patients with changes in mental status characterized by delirium, obtundation or stupor should be immediately evaluated for meningitis by examination of the cerebrospinal fluid. If the findings are normal and typhoid fever is suspected, adults and children should imme-diately be treated with high-dose intravenous dexamethasone in addition to antimicrobials. Dexamethasone, given in an initial dose of 3 mg/kg body weight by slow intravenous infusion over 30 minutes, followed 6 hours later by 1 mg per kg body weight every 6 hours for a total of eight times, can reduce mortality by approximately 80–90% in these high-risk patients. Dexamethasone, given in a lower dose, is not effective. High-dose steroid treatment need not await the results of typhoid blood cultures if other causes of severe disease are unlikely.

Prevention and control measures

- Health education, clean water, food inspection, proper food handling and proper sewage disposal are essential in preventing typhoid fever outbreaks.

- Early detection and containment of the cases are paramount in reducing dissemination. The health authorities must be informed if one or more

---

[7] Of the available fluoroquinolones, ofloxacin, ciprofloxacin, fleroxacin and perfloxacin are all highly active and equivalent in efficacy. Nalidixic acid and norfloxacin do not achieve adequate blood concentrations and should not be used in typhoid fever.

suspected cases are identified. The outbreak should be confirmed following WHO guidelines, and a referral laboratory should be consulted whenever possible to quickly obtain an antimicrobial sensitivity pattern of the outbreak strain.

Vaccination

- The old parenteral, killed, whole-cell vaccine was effective but produced an unacceptable rate of side-effects. Nowadays, a parenteral vaccine containing the polysaccharide Vi antigen is the vaccine of choice in displaced populations. A live oral vaccine using *S.* Typhi strain Ty21a is also available. Neither the polysaccharide vaccine nor the Ty21a vaccine is licensed for children under 2 years of age. The Ty21a vaccine should not be used in patients receiving antimicrobials.

- Mass vaccination may be an adjunct for the control of typhoid fever during a sustained, high-incidence epidemic. This is especially true when access to well functioning medical services is not possible or in the case of a multidrug-resistant strain. If the involved community cannot be fully vaccinated, children aged 2–19 years should be given priority.

5.21 Typhus (epidemic louse-borne)

Basic facts

- Typhus is a rickettsial disease caused by the pathogen *Rickettsia prowazeki*.
- It is transmitted by the human body louse, which is infected by feeding on the blood of a patient with acute typhus. Infected lice excrete rickettsiae in their faeces, and humans are infected by rubbing faeces or crushed lice into the bite.
- The disease is endemic in the highlands and cold areas of Africa, Asia and South America. Cases occurred in the past in the Balkans and parts of the former Soviet Union, and cases of Brill-Zinsser disease (recrudescent typhus) are still reported from these regions.
- Refugees and displaced persons in affected areas are at a high risk of epidemics if there are overcrowding, poor washing facilities and body lice.
- Large outbreaks have been reported among refugees in Burundi, Ethiopia and Rwanda.
- The crude mortality rate ranges from 10% to 40% without treatment, and can rise to 50% in the elderly.
- The crude mortality rate is around 70% among those who develop complications.

Clinical features

- The incubation period is 1–2 weeks, commonly 12 days.
- There is a sudden onset of fever, chills, headache and generalized pain.
- A macular rash spreads over the trunk and limbs after 5–6 days of the illness.

- In severe cases, complications such as vascular collapse, gangrene, acute respiratory distress syndrome and coma can occur.

Diagnosis

- Typhus has a nonspecific clinical presentation, so laboratory testing is usually needed to confirm the diagnosis for the first cases in a suspected epidemic.
- Serological techniques are used, the most common being the indirect fluorescent antibody test.
- Other tests are the enzyme-linked immunosorbent assay and complement fixation.
- Only initial cases should be confirmed; after confirmation of an epidemic the diagnosis should be clinical.

Case management

- In areas where typhus is known to present a risk, all newly arrived refugees or internally displaced persons in a camp or community should be screened and, if body lice are found, mass delousing should be carried out.
- Prompt treatment of patients with antimicrobials is essential.
- The treatment of first choice is a single oral dose of doxycycline (5 mg/kg body weight).
- Typhus can also be treated with tetracycline or chloramphenicol orally with a loading dose of 2–3 g (in children, tetracycline at 25–50 mg/kg body weight, chloramphenicol 50 mg/kg body weight), followed by daily doses of 1–2 g/day in four divided doses at 6-hour intervals until the patient becomes afebrile (usually 3–7 days) plus one day.
- In severe cases, patients should be admitted to hospital and given intravenous tetracycline or chloramphenicol.

Prevention and control measures

- Once an epidemic is confirmed, all patients and contacts should be deloused using permethrin powder 0.5%. Permethrin is applied to all clothes and bedding using a shaker-top container or a special hand-held powder duster. The powder is blown into the clothing through the neck openings, up the sleeves, up the legs and from all sides of the loosened waist. If this is not available a 25% solution of benzyl benzoate (found in all essential drug kits) can be applied and washed off 24 hours later.
- Clothing and bedding that have not been used should also be treated. One easy method is to place all clothing and bedclothes in a blanket, add dusting powder and shake. Alternatively, such items can be impregnated with permethrin by the same methods as are used for impregnating mosquito nets. Clothing thus treated will retain its insecticidal properties for several washes and will resist re-infestation by lice.

5.22 Viral haemorrhagic fevers (VHF)

Basic facts

Viruses causing haemorrhagic fevers (HF) belong to different taxonomic groups and are characterized by different modes of transmission, geographical distribution, disease severity and different propensity to cause haemorrhagic signs in those who are infected (Table 5.17). HF viruses include some of the most frequently lethal infectious agents, and some of them can be highly transmissible by direct contact from person to person, resulting in community outbreaks or nosocomial transmission.

The incubation period is usually 5–10 days (range 2–21 days), with the exception of haemorrhagic fever with renal syndrome (HFRS, caused by Hantaan virus) in which symptoms appear on average 2–3 weeks after infection.

Depending on the area at risk and the infectious agent involved, disasters and war conditions may increase the risk of HF occurrence through different circumstances: contact with rodents (HFRS, Lassa fever, New World VHF), contact with carcasses of wild infected animals (Ebola HF, Crimean-Congo HF) or breakdown of mosquito control programmes (yellow fever, dengue, Rift Valley fever). Moreover, the poor condition of many health care facilities frequently seen in emergency-affected countries increases the risk of nosocomial outbreaks of VHF agents transmitted by blood or fomites, particularly with the lack of minimal barrier nursing procedures, the lack of safe disposal of sharps and the reuse of infected needles and syringes.

Table 5.17   **Some features of the main agents of viral haemorrhagic fevers**

Family	Disease	Vector in nature	Geographical distribution	Mortality	Risk of person-to-person transmission and nosocomial outbreaks
Filoviridae	Ebola HF, Marburg HF	Unknown [a]	Equatorial Africa	50–90% (Ebola HF), 23–70% (Marburg HF)	Yes
Arenaviridae	Lassa fever	Rodent	West Africa	15–20%	Yes
	New World VHF [b]	Rodent	Americas	15–30%	Yes
Bunyaviridae	Crimean-Congo HF	Tick	Africa, central Asia, eastern Europe, Middle East	20–50%	Yes
	Rift Valley fever	Mosquito	Africa, Arabic peninsula	< 1%	No
	Haemorrhagic fever with renal syndrome	Rodent	Asia, Balkans, Europe, Eurasia	1–15%	No
Flaviviridae	Dengue fever, dengue HF, dengue shock syndrome (see Section 5.5)	Mosquito	Asia, Africa, Pacific, Americas	< 1%	No
	Yellow fever (see Section 5.23)	Mosquito	Africa, tropical Americas	20%	No

[a] Contact with infected apes through hunting activities or consumption of ape meat has been the origin of several outbreaks.
[b] Argentine, Bolivian, Brazilian and Venezuelan haemorrhagic fevers.

Clinical features

Initial symptoms of VHF are not specific and overlap with the clinical presentation of more common infectious diseases seen in endemic areas: fever, headache, back pain, myalgias, nausea, vomiting, diarrhoea, prostration and conjunctival injection.

More specific signs (maculopapular rash with filoviruses, severe pharyngitis with Lassa fever, jaundice with Rift Valley fever) are inconsistent or difficult to assess under field conditions.

Haemorrhages (petechiae, nosebleeds, bleeding gums, ecchymosis, melaena, haematemesis, bloody diarrhoea) are by definition the distinguishing feature of VHF, but they are not always present, even in the late stages of the disease. The combination of compatible clinical symptoms, endemic area and clustered cases is essential to suspect an outbreak of VHF (see WHO case definition, Annex 5).

When isolated patients present with fever and haemorrhagic signs outside of an outbreak situation, standard barrier nursing procedures must be reinforced. Nevertheless, more common diseases are likely to be the cause (e.g. malaria or typhoid fever complicated with disseminated intravascular coagulation).

Diagnosis

Depending on the circumstances of sampling and on the causal agent, laboratory confirmation of VHF can be based on:

- antigen or antibody detection in serum,
- polymerase chain reaction from any infected sample,
- virus isolation, or
- immunohistochemical staining of autopsy material.

This last method has been shown to allow the retrospective diagnosis of filovirus infection from dead bodies, and a relatively safe procedure has been developed for sampling and shipment of diagnostic skin snips in fixative solution.

Any other method involving the manipulation, shipment and analysis of material potentially infected with VHF agents should follow strict biosafety procedures. As soon as one case of VHF is suspected, contact should be made with public health officers, and ultimately with WHO representatives, in order to organize an appropriate outbreak response, including collection/shipment of diagnostic material under safe conditions to a reference laboratory.

Case management

In most cases of VHF there is no specific treatment, but some general principles of case management must be followed.

- As long as diagnosis of VHF is not confirmed, consider and treat for more common and potentially confounding diseases, in particular malaria, typhoid fever, louse-borne typhus, relapsing fever or leptospirosis.
- Avoid nosocomial transmission by strict implementation of barrier nursing. If barrier nursing material is not available and a highly transmissible form of VHF is likely, avoid any invasive procedure (e.g. blood sampling, injections, placement of infusion lines or nasogastric tubes) and put on at least one layer of gloves for any direct contact with the patient.
- Supportive treatment – analgesic drugs (excluding aspirin and non-steroidal anti-inflammatories), fluid replacement or antimicrobial therapy if secondary infection is suspected – can make a difference, at least in the comfort of the patient. In the case of HFRS, dengue HF and dengue shock syndrome, proper management of fluid and electrolyte balance can be life-saving.

- Ribavirin (ideally given intravenously) improves the prognosis dramatically if given early in Lassa fever episodes, and probably also in cases of Crimean-Congo HF, HFRS and some New World HF.

Prevention and control measures

Where outbreaks of VHF are known to occur, routine prevention measures should include reinforced sanitation, hospital infection control, case detection and health education. In addition, there are specific interventions that can be implemented either to prevent outbreaks or to limit the extension of an established outbreak (Table 5.18). Commercial vaccines against VHF are not available except for yellow fever, where mass vaccination is the mainstay of epidemic control (see Section 5.5).

In the case of an outbreak, population movements can contribute to the spread of infection to non-affected areas. Contacts under daily follow-up should be encouraged to limit their movements.

Table 5.18   **Specific interventions to prevent or limit disease outbreaks**

Disease	Specific preventive measures	Control measures/outbreak
Ebola HF, Marburg HF		Strict barrier nursing in suspected/confirmed cases
Lassa fever	Rodent control	
New World VHF	Rodent control	
Crimean-Congo HF	Avoidance of contact with tick-infested animals	
Rift Valley fever	Mosquito control	Mosquito control
Haemorrhagic fever with renal syndrome	Avoidance of contact with rodents	Rodent control
Dengue fever, dengue HF, and dengue shock syndrome (see Section 5.6)	Mosquito control (see Sections 2.4.1 and 2.4.2)	Mosquito control
Yellow fever (see Section 5.23)	Mosquito control (see Sections 2.4.1 and 2.4.2)	Mass vaccination plus mosquito control

Barrier nursing

To prevent secondary infections, contact with the patient's lesions and body fluids should be minimized using standard isolation precautions:

- isolation of patients,
- restriction of access to patients' wards,
- use of protective clothing,
- safe disposal of waste,
- disinfection of reusable supplies and equipment,
- safe funeral practices.

Simple guidelines have been developed (see selected reading below) on how to implement these principles, even where resources are limited.

Further reading

Infection control for viral haemorrhagic fevers in the African health care setting. Geneva, World Health Organization, 1998 (document WHO/EMC/ESR/98.2).

5.23 Yellow fever

Basic facts

- Yellow fever is an acute infectious disease caused by a flavivirus.
- Mild cases are clinically indeterminate but severe cases are characterized by jaundice.
- Overall case-fatality rates are around 5%, but among those with jaundice they are 20–50%.
- The disease is found in Africa and South America.
- There has been a dramatic increase in the incidence of the disease in the past 15 years.
- Yellow fever has two types of transmission cycle: jungle and urban. In the jungle cycle, the virus is transmitted among non-human primates by different mosquito vectors; humans are only incidentally infected. In the urban cycle, the virus is transmitted from infected humans to susceptible humans by *Aedes aegypti* mosquitoes, which breed in household containers and refuse.

Clinical features

- The incubation period is usually 3–6 days.
- An *acute phase* lasting for 2 to 5 days with:
  - a sudden onset of fever,
  - headache or backache,
  - muscle pain,
  - nausea,
  - vomiting,
  - red eyes (injected conjunctiva).

  This phase of yellow fever can be confused with other diseases that also present with fever, headache, nausea and vomiting because jaundice may not be present in less severe (or mild) cases of yellow fever. The less severe cases are often non-fatal.
- A temporary *period of remission* follows the acute phase in 5–20% of cases.

- After this brief remission, a *toxic phase* can follow with jaundice within 2 weeks of onset of first symptoms. Haemorrhagic manifestations (bleeding from the gums, nose or in the stool, vomiting blood) and signs of renal failure may occur.

WHO case definition for yellow fever surveillance:

Suspected case: An illness characterized by an acute onset of fever followed by jaundice within 2 weeks of onset of the first symptoms AND one of the following: bleeding from the nose, gums, skin, or gastrointestinal tract OR death within 3 weeks of the onset of illness.

Confirmed case: A suspected case that is confirmed by laboratory results or linked to another confirmed case or outbreak.

Outbreak: An outbreak of yellow fever is at least one confirmed case.

Diagnosis

- Diagnosis of the disease is through serology. Two blood samples must be sent to a reference laboratory for confirmation.

Case management

- Supportive treatment should be given – no specific treatment is available for yellow fever.
- In the toxic phase, supportive treatment includes therapies for dehydration and fever. In severe cases, death can occur between the 7th and 10th day after onset of the first symptoms.
- For fever: give paracetamol.
- For dehydration: give oral rehydration salts or IV fluids depending on the assessment of dehydration.
- For restlessness: give diazepam.
- For malaria: give an antimalarial recommended for your area.
- For bacterial infections: give antibacterials recommended for your area.
- Access by daytime-biting mosquitoes should be prevented by screening the patient or using a bednet.

Prevention and control measures

- Exposure to mosquitoes should be avoided, including the use of protective clothing and repellents.
- Sleeping and living quarters should be screened.
- A very effective vaccine is available, and mass vaccination is a key intervention for outbreak control (see Section 2.6.7).
- In urban areas, mosquito breeding sites should be destroyed.

Further reading

District guidelines for yellow fever surveillance. Geneva, World health Organization, 1998 (document WHO/EPI/GEN/98.09).

Vainio J, Cutts F. *Yellow fever*. Geneva, World health Organization, 1998 (document WHO/EPI/GEN/98.11).

WHO report on global surveillance of epidemic-prone infectious diseases. Chapter 2. Yellow fever. Geneva, World Health Organization, 2000 (document WHO/CDS/CSR/ISR/2000.1).

Yellow fever – Technical Consensus Meeting, Geneva, 2–3 March 1998. Geneva, World health Organization, 1998. (document WHO/EPI/GEN/98.08).

ANNEXES

1. WHO reference values for emergencies

Table A1.1   **Cut-off values for emergency warning**

Health status	More than
Daily crude mortality rate	1 per 10 000 population
Daily under-5 mortality rate	2 per 10 000 children under 5

Table A1.2   **Basic needs**

Water	Average requirements
Quantity	20 litres per person per day
Quality	250 people per water point *not more than 150 metres from housing*
Sanitation	
Latrine	Ideally 1 per family Minimum 1 seat per 20 people *30 metres from housing*
Refuse disposal	1 communal pit per 500 people *2 x 5 x 2 metres*
Shelter	
Individual requirements	3.5 square metres per person
Collective requirements	30 square metres per person *including shelter, sanitation, services, warehousing, access*
Household fuel	
Firewood	15 kg per household per day *with one economic stove per family, the needs may be* *reduced to 5 kg per stove per day*

Table A1.3   **Health care needs**

Predicted morbidity	Expected attack rate in emergency situations
Acute respiratory infections, < 5 years	10% per month in cold weather
Diarrhoeal diseases, < 5 years	50% per month
Malaria, non-immune population	50% per month
Essential primary health care activities	**Target**
Under-5 clinic and growth monitoring	all children aged 0–59 months
Antenatal clinic	all pregnancies
Assisted deliveries	all deliveries
Vaccination	**Target**
Tetanus toxoid	all deliveries
BCG	all newborns
DPT1-TT1	all children aged 0–1 year
DPT2-TT2	all children aged 0–1 year
DPT3	all children aged 0–1 year
Measles	all children aged 9–12 months

Table A1.4   **Health personnel requirements**

Activity	Output of 1 person per hour
Vaccination	30 vaccinations
Under-5 clinic and growth monitoring	10 children
Antenatal clinic	6 women
Assisted delivery	1 delivery
OPD[a] consultation	6 consultations
OPD[a] treatments, e.g. dressings	6 treatments
Health worker requirements	60 staff per 10 000 population

[a] *OPD: outpatient department*
   Note: 1 person per day = 7 hours of field work.

Table A1.5   **Health supply requirements**

Essential drugs and medical equipment	
WHO Basic Emergency Kit	1 kit for 10 000 population for 3 months
WHO Supplementary Emergency Kit	1 kit for 10 000 population for 3 months
Safe water	
Preparing 1 litre of stock solution	Calcium hypochlorite 70%: 15 g/litre water **or** bleaching powder 30%: 33 g/litre water **or** sodium hypochlorite 5%: 250 ml/litre water **or** sodium hypochlorite 10%: 110 ml/litre water
Using the stock solution	0.6 ml or three drops/litre water 60 ml/100 litres water

Note: allow the chlorinated water to stand at least 30 minutes before using.

2. Health assessment – sample survey forms

2A. RAPID HEALTH ASSESSMENT

Date of visit: ____	____	____ (dd mm yyyy)	Compiled by:	Organization:
Name of location:	Urban / Rural (circle one)	Province/Governorate:
District/Area and subdistrict:	Name of town or city:	Quarter/Neighbourhood:
Reference code:	Other location information:	

1. Access

Routes to location: _____ _____ ____   Distance from nearest airfield? _____ km

Distance from hard surface road? _____ km   Routes passable with lorry: Yes / No

Are there security problems? Yes / No – If yes, specify, providing the source: _____ _____

_____

Other information about access: _____

_____

Telephones working? Yes / No – If yes, can call: locally / capital / international

2. Population

Source of information: Name: _____ Title: _____

Total population (approximate or estimate): _____ Number of displaced people: _____

Estimated sex ratio of current adult population: _____ % women

Estimated number of children < 5 years: _____ **OR** estimated % of total population < 5 years _____

Estimated number of pregnant women: _____

Are there other especially vulnerable population groups in the area (for example, in institutions):

_____

3. Main health concerns

What are the main health concerns currently?

As reported by the population: _____

As reported by health staff: _____

_____

4. Death rates in recent time period (days, weeks or months)

Source of information: Name: _____ Title: _____

Overall mortality rate (all ages): _____ deaths per _____ persons per _____ (recent time period)

Mortality rate in children < 5: _____ deaths per _____ children < 5 years per _____ (recent time period)

5. Health facilities

Source of information: Name: _____ Title: _____

No. of hospitals in this area: _____ No. of primary health centers (with doctor)_____

No. of primary health centres (without doctor): _____ No. of private clinics: _____

No. of other health facilities in this area: _____
(fill out tables below with description of individual health facilities)

If no hospitals in the area, where are patients referred for specialized medical/surgical care?

_____

Is there an ambulance service: Yes / No

    If yes, how many working ambulances? _____

Have the health facilities been looted? Yes / No

    If yes, what medical equipment has been stolen/destroyed? _____

_____

6. Maternal and child health and nutrition

Source of information: Name: _____ Title: _____

Is there access to an emergency obstetric care centre in the area assessed? Yes / No

    If yes, which? _____

    If no, where is the closest one? _____

What % of children 1–4 years of age have been vaccinated for measles: _____ %

Is there a community child care unit in this location: Yes (No._____) / No

    If yes, how many children are enrolled in all units? _____

Is there a therapeutic feeding centre? Yes (No._____) / No

    If yes, how many children enrolled? _____

Has there been a recent assessment of malnutrition in this location? Yes / No

    If yes, prevalence of acute malnutrition: _____ %

How measured? Weight-for-age / Weight-for-height / MUAC / Other_____

7. Outbreaks of disease

Have there been any infectious disease outbreaks (unusual numbers of cases) in recent days/weeks?

If yes, describe symptoms, place, number of people affected: _____

_____

8. Mine/UXO injuries

Have there been any injuries in recent months from mines or unexploded ordnance: Yes / No

If yes, describe and identify location: **(Do not visit the location!)** _____

_____

9. Other health problems/issues

_____

_____

10. Basic description of health facilities. Name of contact and contact information:

No.	Name of health facility	Type of facility	MoH or other (specify)?	Functioning (fully, partially, not at all)	Level of damage (use HIC codes on next page)	No. total beds		Average No. outpatients seen per day		No. maternity beds		Average No. deliveries attended during one week	
						Total	Occupied today	6 months ago	Today	6 months ago	Today	6 months ago	Today
1													
2													
3													
4													
5													

No.	Name of health facility	No. doctors		No. nurses		No. other professional staff	
		6 months ago	Today	6 months ago	Today	6 months ago	Today
1							
2							
3							
4							
5							

11. Availability of drugs, equipment, and utilities

No.	Amoxicillin Co-trimox. Ampicillin	ORS	Anti-malarial drugs	IV fluids	Other	Food for patients or malnourished	Electricity (if no, what is lacking?)	Water supply (if no, what is lacking?)	Toilet (if no, what is lacking?)	No. operating theatres	Vaccine cold chain	Other expressed needs (attach list if necessary)
1												
2												
3												
4												
5												

(see Table A1 below for more details on drugs and equipment)

Codes for infrastructure damage assessment:

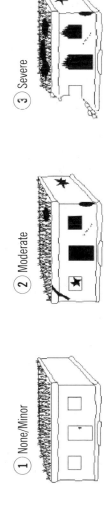

(1) None/Minor

(2) Moderate

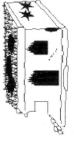

(3) Severe

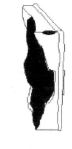

(4) Destroyed

12. Review of outpatient register

Health facility: _____ Type of facility: _____

Time period (collect data of a recent period, preferably of the week preceding the visit)

Beginning date: _____ Ending date: _____

Diagnosis of outpatients	< 5 years	5+ years	Total
Acute lower respiratory infection			
Acute watery diarrhoea (including cholera)			
Bloody diarrhoea (dysentery)			
Measles			
Meningitis			
Malaria			
Acute jaundice syndrome			
Acute haemorrhagic fever syndrome			
War injury			
Injury (not war-related)			
Malnutrition			
TB new cases (with/without lab. confirmation)			
Diabetes			
Cardiovascular disease			
Other/unknown			
Total consultations during time period			

13. Review of death register

Health facility or data source: _____

Time period (collect data of a recent period, preferably of the two weeks, or more, preceding the visit)

Beginning date: _____ Ending date: _____

Cause of death	< 5 years	5+ years	Total
Acute lower respiratory infection			
Acute watery diarrhoea (including cholera)			
Bloody diarrhoea (dysentery)			
Measles			
Meningitis			
Malaria			

Cause of death	< 5 years	5+ years	Total
Acute jaundice syndrome			
Acute haemorrhagic fever syndrome			
War injury			
Injury (not war-related)			
Cardiovascular			
Respiratory			
Cancer			
Maternal death			
Other/unknown			
Total deaths			

14. Recommendations for immediate public health action

What must be put in place *immediately* to reduce avoidable mortality and morbidity?

_____

_____

_____

Which activities must be implemented for this to happen?

_____

_____

_____

What are the risks to be monitored?

_____

_____

_____

How can we monitor them?

_____

_____

_____

Which inputs are needed to implement all this?

_____

_____

_____

Table A1   **More detailed list of drugs and equipment**

List of key drugs and equipment for CLINICS; if possible try to verify stock quantity and duration of availability

Name of health facility: _____ Type of facility: _____

		Health facility				
Disease	**Selected drugs**	**1**	**2**	**3**	**4**	**5**
Diarrhoea	Oral rehydration salts Co-trimoxazole tablets					
ARI	Co-trimoxazole tablets Procaine penicillin injection Paediatric paracetamol tablets					
Malaria	Chloroquine tablets SP Quinine Artesunate Amodiaquine					
Anaemia	Ferrous salt + folic acid tablets					
Worm infestations	Mebendazole tablets Albendazole					
Conjunctivitis	Tetracycline eye ointment					
Skin infections	Iodine, gentian violet or local alternative					
Fungal skin infections	Benzoic acid + salicylic acid ointment					
Scabies and others	Benzyl benzoate lotion Soap Zinc oxide ointment Permethrin/malathion					
Pain	Acetylsalicylic acid or paracetamol tablets					
Prophylactic drugs	Retinol (vitamin A) Ferrous salt + folic acid tablets					
Vaccine-preventable diseases	Intact cold chain Syringes and needles BCG vaccine/adjuvant Measles vaccine DPT vaccine Polio vaccine					
Nutrition	Height board Scale High-protein biscuits Other supplemental feeding food Therapeutic milk (F-75 & F-100)					

List of additional key drugs and equipment for FIRST-LEVEL HOSPITAL; if possible try to verify stock quantity and duration of availability

Name of health facility: _____ Type of facility: _____

		Health facility				
Disease	**Selected drugs**	**1**	**2**	**3**	**4**	**5**
Trauma/ surgery	General anaesthetics (ketamine, thiopental)					
	Local anaesthetics					
	Preoperative medication and sedation for short-term procedures (atropine, diazepam)					
	Parenteral solutions for rehydration + giving set + canulae: − ringer's lactate − glucose 5%					
	Blood substitutes/transfusions					
	Muscle relaxants, cholinesterase inhibitors					
Pain	Non-opioids (ASS, ibuprofen, paracetamol)					
	Opioid analgesicss (morphine, pethidine)					
Allergies, anaphylactic reactions	Adrenaline (epinephrine) inj.					
	Hydrocortisone powder for inj.					
	Prednisolone tablets					
Convulsions	Phenobarbital tablets					
	Phenytoin tablets					
Infections	Amoxicillin tablets					
	Ampicillin powder for inj.					
	Benzylpenicillin powder inj.					
	Cloxacillin powder Inj.					
	Co-trimoxazole tablets					
	Phenoxymethylpenicillin tablets					
	Procaine benzylpenicillin tablets					
	Chloramphenicol capsules					
	Doxycycline capsules, tablets					
	Erythromycin tablets					
	Gentamicin injection					
	Metronidazole tablet					
	Trimethoprim + sulfamethoxazole					
	Tetracycline eye ointment					
	Gentamicin eye drops					

Disease	Selected drugs	Health facility				
		1	2	3	4	5
Hypertension, coronary heart disease	Atenolol tablets Hydralazine powder for injection Methyldopa tablets Nitroglycerin tablets Furosemide injection Hydrochlorothiazide tablet					
Disinfectant, antiseptics	Chlorhexidine solution Polyvidone iodine solution Silver sulfazidine cream Chlorine-based compound					
Diabetes	Oral antidiabetics Insulins					
Obstetrics	Caesarian equipment Equipment for assisted delivery Ergometrine tablets, injection Oxytocin injection					
Psychotic disorders	Chlorpromazine tablets, injections					
Asthma	Aminophylline injection Salbutamol tablet/aerosol Beclometasone aerosol Ipratropium bromine aerosol Adrenaline injection					
Hormonal contraceptives	Ethinylestradiol + levonorgestrel tablet Levonorgestrel tablet Medroxyprogesterone acetate depot injection					

Expressed needs for specific drugs and equipment

Source of information: Name: _____ Title: _____

Drugs and equipment needed:

_____

_____

_____

_____

_____

Table A2 **To be considered if the health assessment relates to IDPs/refugees in a camp or housed in public buildings**

Note that this is not intended to be a full assessment of the facilities available for the IDPs/refugees. This should be carried out by the appropriate responsible agencies (see Section 9 of Annex 2B–Health survey). If the IDPs/refugees are already under the care of such an entity the following table should be filled in consultation with them, if considered necessary.

Are the following adequate:	Yes	No	Immediate requirements
Water supply?			
Food distribution? Source?			
Excreta disposal?			
Shelter?			
Soap, buckets, etc. for washing?			
Fuel and cooking utensils?			
Other vital needs?			
Which agency/organization is responsible for:			
– management of the camp (location)?			
– provision of health care?			

2B. HEALTH SURVEY

1. Basic data

RECORD NUMBER: _____

1. Date of study (dd/mm/yyyy): _____ / _____ / _____

2. Section number: _____

3. Name of village/camp/site: _____

4. Date of arrival in area/site (dd/mm/yyyy): _____ / _____ / _____

5. Name of head of household: _____

6. Male- or female-headed household: Male ❑   Female ❑

7. Total number of people in household: _____

8. Total number of children under 5 years: _____

9. Total number of pregnant or lactating women: _____

10. Total number of elderly persons (over 65 years): _____

2. Member information list

Main respondent: ❏ Wife of head of household *and* mother of the children (if there are any children)   ❏ other (specify) _____

Head of the household: ❏ male   ❏ female   ❏ refugee status   ❏ no refugee status

List below all individuals who *since onset of crisis*, are or have been living for at least one month in the household, including those who died or are missing

Household member number	Main respondent (x)	Head of household (x)	Age in **years** (if 2 years or older)	Age in **months** (if under 2 years)	Sex (M/F)	Present at interview? (yes/No)	Household member is: - Core family - Extended family - Other (specify)	Household member is today: 1. Alive, always lived in this household 2. Alive, moved in, still present 3. Alive, moved out 4. Alive in prison 5. Died, had always lived in this household 6. Died, moved in/out 7. Missing/unknown	If dead or missing, since when? (date: dd/mm)
1									/
2									/
3									/
4									/
5									/
6									/
7									/
8									/
9									/
10									/
11									/
12									/

3. Retrospective mortality

Total number of deaths since start of crisis

Death number	Age in **years** (if 2 years or older)	Age in **months** (12 to 23 months)	Age in **months** (under 12 months)	Sex (M/F)	Month of death: 2 = Feb 2003 3 = Mar 2003 4 = Apr 2003 5 = May 2003 6 = Jun 2003 etc.	Cause of death: 1 = watery diarrhoea 2 = bloody diarrhoea 3 = measles 4 = cough ± difficulty breathing 5 = fever of unknown origin 6 = trauma/injury i.e. 6(a) = mine/ UXO*, 6(b) = war-related other than mine/UXO, 6(c) = road traffic accident, or 6(d) = other 7 = death during or right after childbirth 8 = other (specify)
1						
2						
3						
4						
5						
6						
7						
8						
9						
10						
11						
12						

* *Unexploded ordnance*

4. Nutritional status and vaccination coverage of children under 5 years

Household member number	Sex (M/F)	Age (in months)	Weight (in kg, precision to 100 g)	Length or height (in cm, precision to 0.5 cm)	Presence of bilateral pitting oedema (Yes/No)	Date of measles vaccination (card) (Yes/No)	OPV (all 4 doses at appropriate time intervals) vaccination (card) (Yes/No)	DPT (all 4 doses at appropriate time intervals) or DT vaccination (card) (Yes/No)
1								
2								
3								
4								
5								
6								
7								
8								
9								
10								
11								
12								

5. Communicable diseases in children under five years (ALRI, diarrhoea, measles)

In the last 2 weeks, has any child under 5 years of age in the household suffered from a cough or cold, diarrhoea or any fever?   ☐ Yes   ☐ No

If Yes, complete table – If No, cross out table

Household number	Number of episodes of:				Did you access medical assistance during any episode? (Yes/No)	If accessed medical assistance, at what level? 1. Traditional healer 2. Community health worker 3. Health centre 4. Hospital (Mark option with cross)	Did you receive medications? (Yes/No)	If received medications, what were they? 1. Antimicrobial 2. ORS 3. Other/unknown (Mark option with cross)
	Fever (e.g. suspected malaria)	Cough with fever (± difficult breathing)	Rash with fever	Diarrhoea				
1						1. 2. 3. 4.		1. 2. 3.
2						1. 2. 3. 4.		1. 2. 3.
3						1. 2. 3. 4.		1. 2. 3.
4						1. 2. 3. 4.		1. 2. 3.
5						1. 2. 3. 4.		1. 2. 3.
6						1. 2. 3. 4.		1. 2. 3.
7						1. 2. 3. 4.		1. 2. 3.
8						1. 2. 3. 4.		1. 2. 3.
9						1. 2. 3. 4.		1. 2. 3.
10						1. 2. 3. 4.		1. 2. 3.
11						1. 2. 3. 4.		1. 2. 3.
12						1. 2. 3. 4.		1. 2. 3.

6. Noncommunicable diseases (hypertension, diabetes mellitus, heart disease and cancer)

Since crisis:

– has there been anyone in the household with **high blood pressure** *(diagnosed by a physician)*? ☐ Yes ☐ No

– anyone in the household with **diabetes** *(diagnosed by a physician)*? ☐ Yes ☐ No

– anyone in the household with **heart disease** *(diagnosed by a physician)*? ☐ Yes ☐ No

– anyone in the household with **cancer** *(diagnosed by a physician)*? ☐ Yes ☐ No

If Yes, complete table (one line per person and disease, same person can have more than one disease) – If No, cross out table

Household member number	Disease: 1. Hypertension 2. Diabetes 3. Heart disease 4. Cancer *(one line per person and disease)*	Information source: 1. Health card 2. Self-reported 3. Household member (other than the patient) *(list all sources below)*	Has been or is under regular medical follow-up? (Yes/No)	Any scheduled appointment missed? (Yes/No)		Has been/is on regular drug treatment? (Yes/No)	Interruption in drug treatment of any length? (Yes/No)		As of today, is he/she: 1. Alive, home 2. Alive, in hospital 3. Alive, elsewhere 4. Died, at home 5. Died, in hospital 6. Died, elsewhere
				In the last month	Since (date)		In the last month	Since (date)	
1									
2									
3									
4									
5									
6									
7									
8									
9									
10									
11									
12									

7. Maternal health (antenatal care)

Since crisis, has there been anybody pregnant or become pregnant? ☐ Yes ☐ No

If Yes, complete table – If No, cross out table

Household member number	*Guess how many months since day conceived*	Information source: 1. Antenatal card 2. Self-reported 3. Household member other than the one pregnant *(list all sources below)*	How many times gone for antenatal care? *(Write "zero" if never gone)*	Anti-tetanus vaccination given? + HB + urine check 1. No 2. Yes, verified by card 3. Yes, reported orally	Asked to attend more than one check per month? (Yes/No)	If *Yes*, always gone? (Yes/No)	If *No*, rank up to 3 reasons	Admitted to hospital during pregnancy to ensure adequate follow-up? (Yes/No)	Any medicine prescribed during pregnancy? (Yes/No)	If *Yes*, was/is it possible to complete the treatment? (Yes/No)	If *No*, rank up to 3 reasons
1							1. 2. 3.				1. 2. 3.
2							1. 2. 3.				1. 2. 3.
3							1. 2. 3.				1. 2. 3.
4							1. 2. 3.				1. 2. 3.
5							1. 2. 3.				1. 2. 3.

8. Maternal health (delivery / stillbirth / abortion / post-natal care)

Since crisis, has any woman in the household given birth or lost a child during pregnancy/immediately after childbirth?   ☐ Yes   ☐ No

If Yes, complete table – If No, cross out table

Household member number	Baby born: 1. Alive, weight more than 2500 g 2. Alive, weight less than 2500 g 3. Alive, weight not known 4. Dead, born after 28th week 5. Baby lost before end of 28th week	Date conceived (dd/mm) (if not known exactly, make best guess)	Date of delivery or loss of baby (dd/mm) (if not known exactly, make best guess)	Baby born through: 1. Normal (vaginal) delivery or abort 2. Caesarean section	Where did the delivery (or loss of baby) take place? 1. Home 2. MCH 3. PHC 4. Hospital 5. On the way to hospital 6. Other (specify) (e.g. ambulance, private transport)	If at MCH, PHC or Hospital, how long did it take to get there? 1. 1 hour or less 2. 1–2 hours 3. 2–4 hours 4. more than 4 hours	If home delivery was it own choice? (Yes/No)	If No, rank up to 3 reasons	If home delivery, assisted by whom? 1. Nobody 2. Family/friend 3. Nurse 4. Midwife 5. Doctor 6. TBA	Gone for any post-natal care visit? (Yes/No)
1								1. 2. 3.		
2								1. 2. 3.		
3								1. 2. 3.		
4								1. 2. 3.		
5								1. 2. 3.		

9. Environment

Shelter

1. Type of habitation (circle):   1   2   3   4 (specify) _____

   1 = plastic roof only; 2 = simple hut; 3 = tent; 4 = other

Sanitation

2. Latrines (circle):   1   2   3   4   5   6 (specify) _____

   1 = one latrine/toilet per household; 2 = collective latrines; 3 = trench; 4 = defecation field; 5 = no specific area; 6 = other

Water

3. Distance from public tap/water point: _____ m

4. Head of household has knowledge about use of disinfected water: ☐ Yes ☐ No

5. Number of water containers (20 litres) per household (e.g. ? for 10 litres): _____

6. Number of times water containers filled per day: _____

7. Availability of washing and bathing facilities: ☐ Yes ☐ No

8. Presence of stagnant water near house: ☐ Yes ☐ No

Non-food items

9. Number of blankets in household: _____

10. Adequate clothing (at least one change of clothes, adapted to climate): ☐ Yes ☐ No

11. Adequate amount of fuel and cooking pots: ☐ Yes ☐ No

Refuse

12. Refuse disposal method (circle):   1   2   3   4   5 (specify) _____

   1 = designated communal pits; 2 = haphazard piling; 3 = household pit; 4 = no specific area; 5 = other

3. NCHS/WHO normalized reference values for weight for height by sex

Weight-for-length (49–84 cm) and weight-for-height (85–110 cm)

Boys' weight (kg)						Girls' weight (kg)				
−4 SD	−3 SD	−2 SD	−1 SD	Median	Length	Median	−1 SD	−2 SD	−3 SD	−4 SD
60%	70%	80%	90%		(cm)		90%	80%	70%	60%
1.8	2.1	2.5	2.8	3.1	49	3.3	2.9	2.6	2.2	1.8
1.8	2.2	2.5	2.9	3.3	50	3.4	3	2.6	2.3	1.9
1.8	2.2	2.6	3.1	3.5	51	3.5	3.1	2.7	2.3	1.9
1.9	2.3	2.8	3.2	3.7	52	3.7	3.3	2.8	2.4	2
1.9	2.4	2.9	3.4	3.9	53	3.9	3.4	3	2.5	2.1
2	2.6	3.1	3.6	4.1	54	4.1	3.6	3.1	2.7	2.2
2.2	2.7	3.3	3.8	4.3	55	4.3	3.8	3.3	2.8	2.3
2.3	2.9	3.5	4	4.6	56	4.5	4	3.5	3	2.4
2.5	3.1	3.7	4.3	4.8	57	4.8	4.2	3.7	3.1	2.6
2.7	3.3	3.9	4.5	5.1	58	5	4.4	3.9	3.3	2.7
2.9	3.5	4.1	4.8	5.4	59	5.3	4.7	4.1	3.5	2.9
3.1	3.7	4.4	5	5.7	60	5.5	4.9	4.3	3.7	3.1
3.3	4	4.6	5.3	5.9	61	5.8	5.2	4.6	3.9	3.3
3.5	4.2	4.9	5.6	6.2	62	6.1	5.4	4.8	4.1	3.5
3.8	4.5	5.2	5.8	6.5	63	6.4	5.7	5	4.4	3.7
4	4.7	5.4	6.1	6.8	64	6.7	6	5.3	4.6	3.9
4.3	5	5.7	6.4	7.1	65	7	6.3	5.5	4.8	4.1
4.5	5.3	6	6.7	7.4	66	7.3	6.5	5.8	5.1	4.3
4.8	5.5	6.2	7	7.7	67	7.5	6.8	6	5.3	4.5
5.1	5.8	6.5	7.3	8	68	7.8	7.1	6.3	5.5	4.8
5.3	6	6.8	7.5	8.3	69	8.1	7.3	6.5	5.8	5
5.5	6.3	7	7.8	8.5	70	8.4	7.6	6.8	6	5.2
5.8	6.5	7.3	8.1	8.8	71	8.6	7.8	7	6.2	5.4
6	6.8	7.5	8.3	9.1	72	8.9	8.1	7.2	6.4	5.6
6.2	7	7.8	8.6	9.3	73	9.1	8.3	7.5	6.6	5.8
6.4	7.2	8	8.8	9.6	74	9.4	8.5	7.7	6.8	6
6.6	7.4	8.2	9	9.8	75	9.6	8.7	7.9	7	6.2
6.8	7.6	8.4	9.2	10	76	9.8	8.9	8.1	7.2	6.4
7	7.8	8.6	9.4	10.3	77	10	9.1	8.3	7.4	6.6
7.1	8	8.8	9.7	10.5	78	10.2	9.3	8.5	7.6	6.7
7.3	8.2	9	9.9	10.7	79	10.4	9.5	8.7	7.8	6.9
7.5	8.3	9.2	10.1	10.9	80	10.6	9.7	8.8	8	7.1
7.6	8.5	9.4	10.2	11.1	81	10.8	9.9	9	8.1	7.2
7.8	8.7	9.6	10.4	11.3	82	11	10.1	9.2	8.3	7.4

Boys' weight (kg)						Girls' weight (kg)				
−4 SD	−3 SD	−2 SD	−1 SD	Median	Length	Median	−1 SD	−2 SD	−3SD	−4 SD
60%	70%	80%	90%		(cm)		90%	80%	70%	60%
7.9	8.8	9.7	10.6	11.5	83	11.2	10.3	9.4	8.5	7.6
8.1	9	9.9	10.8	11.7	84	11.4	10.5	9.6	8.7	7.7
7.8	8.9	9.9	11	12.1	85	11.8	10.8	9.7	8.6	7.6
7.9	9	10.1	11.2	12.3	86	12	11	9.9	8.8	7.7
8.1	9.2	10.3	11.5	12.6	87	12.3	11.2	10.1	9	7.9
8.3	9.4	10.5	11.7	12.8	88	12.5	11.4	10.3	9.2	8.1
8.4	9.6	10.7	11.9	13	89	12.7	11.6	10.5	9.3	8.2
8.6	9.8	10.9	12.1	13.3	90	12.9	11.8	10.7	9.5	8.4
8.8	9.9	11.1	12.3	13.5	91	13.2	12	10.8	9.7	8.5
8.9	10.1	11.3	12.5	13.7	92	13.4	12.2	11	9.9	8.7
9.1	10.3	11.5	12.8	14	93	13.6	12.4	11.2	10	8.8
9.2	10.5	11.7	13	14.2	94	13.9	12.6	11.4	10.2	9
9.4	10.7	11.9	13.2	14.5	95	14.1	12.9	11.6	10.4	9.1
9.6	10.9	12.1	13.4	14.7	96	14.3	13.1	11.8	10.6	9.3
9.7	11	12.4	13.7	15	97	14.6	13.3	12	10.7	9.5
9.9	11.2	12.6	13.9	15.2	98	14.9	13.5	12.2	10.9	9.6
10.1	11.4	12.8	14.1	15.5	99	15.1	13.8	12.4	11.1	9.8
10.3	11.6	13	14.4	15.7	100	15.4	14	12.7	11.3	9.9
10.4	11.8	13.2	14.6	16	101	15.6	14.3	12.9	11.5	10.1
10.6	12	13.4	14.9	16.3	102	15.9	14.5	13.1	11.7	10.3
10.8	12.2	13.7	15.1	16.6	103	16.2	14.7	13.3	11.9	10.5
11	12.4	13.9	15.4	16.9	104	16.5	15	13.5	12.1	10.6
11.2	12.7	14.2	15.6	17.1	105	16.7	15.3	13.8	12.3	10.8
11.4	12.9	14.4	15.9	17.4	106	17	15.5	14	12.5	11
11.6	13.1	14.7	16.2	17.7	107	17.3	15.8	14.3	12.7	11.2
11.8	13.4	14.9	16.5	18	108	17.6	16.1	14.5	13	11.4
12	13.6	15.2	16.8	18.3	109	17.9	16.4	14.8	13.2	11.6
12.2	13.8	15.4	17.1	18.7	110	18.2	16.6	15	13.4	11.9

Notes:

1. Length is generally measured in children below 85 cm, and height in children 85 cm and above. Recumbent length is on average 0.5 cm greater than standing height; although the difference is of no importance to the individual child, a correction may be made by deducting 0.5 cm from all lengths above 84.9 cm if standing height cannot be measured.

2. SD = standard deviation score (or Z-score). The relationship between the percentage of median value and the SD-score or Z-score varies with age and height, particularly in the first year of life, and beyond 5 years. Between 1 and 5 years median −1 SD and median −2 SD correspond to approximately 90% and 80% of median (weight-for-length/height, and weight-for-age), respectively. Beyond 5 years of age or 110 cm (or 100 cm in stunted children) this equivalence is not maintained; median −2 SD is much below 80% of median. Hence the use of "percentage-of-median" is not recommended, particularly in children of school age. Somewhere beyond 10 years or 137 cm, the adolescent growth spurt begins and the time of its onset is variable. The correct interpretation of weight-for-height data beyond this point is therefore difficult.

4. Weekly surveillance report

Guidelines for filling surveillance forms

✔ In each health facility, a daily register of consultations should be kept.

✔ Suggested lay out of register in health facility:

OPD No.	Date	Name	Location	Sex	Date of birth	New case/ follow-up	Diagnosis	Treatment

✔ One person in each health facility should be identified as responsible for data collection and notification of potential epidemics to the Health Coordinator. In each Agency/NGO, one person should be responsible for compiling the data from the daily register for the weekly health report.

✔ The weekly form should be filled out from Monday to Sunday and compiled by the agency/NGO Health Coordinator as soon as possible.

How to fill in the weekly morbidity form

✔ Data should be recorded in two age categories: under 5 years and 5 years and over.

✔ New cases/consultations requested for communicable and noncommunicable diseases.

✔ All cases attending the health facility should be recorded on the Weekly Morbidity Form, including those who are subsequently referred to hospital.

✔ Only the first consultation should be reported; follow-up visits for the same disease should not be reported.

✔ At the end of each week, the reporting officer must count up all the cases and deaths from each disease as recorded in the outpatient and inpatient records. The health worker must select the main cause for the consultation, i.e. one disease/syndrome for each case.

✔ If one of the diseases has epidemic potential marked with an asterisk in the form, record this disease as the main cause of consultation.

✔ "Other communicable diseases" include all cases of communicable diseases not mentioned in the list of diseases eg skin infections

✔ "Other noncommunicable diseases" include all cases of noncommunicable diseases not mentioned in the list of diseases e.g. gastrointestinal problems, heart disease, diabetes.

✔ Diseases of outbreak potential are marked with an asterisk * on the morbidity form. They must be reported to your health coordinator using the *outbreak alert form* if the weekly alert thresholds below are passed (see box on alert thresholds below).

✔ In the event of an increase in the number of cases of a disease/syndrome, surveillance activities may need to be enhanced. For example, active case-finding and case definitions may need to be revised, such as in the event of an outbreak of meningitis.

✔ Record total number of consultations in the health facility in a week.

How to fill in the weekly mortality form:

✔ This form is a line-listing of all deaths.

✔ Fill in all the details as required for each case including names, age, sex, date and location of death and laboratory samples taken, and record a main cause of death for each entry even if "unknown".

✔ Calculations of mortality rates can be performed as follows:

Crude mortality rate (CMR) : Number of deaths for the week/population at the end of the week × 10 000 persons/7 days = deaths/10 000 persons/day. (Alert threshold or AT is 1/10 000/day.)

Under-5 mortality rate (U5MR) : Number of deaths among children <5 years for the week/under 5 year population at the end of the week × 10 000 persons/7 days = deaths/10 000 persons/day (AT is 2/10 000/day).

SAMPLE ALERT THRESHOLDS (may need to be adapted for particular context)

Acute watery diarrhoea:	5 cases in the 5 years and over age group
Bloody diarrhoea:	5 cases
Measles:	1 case
Meningitis – suspected:	5 cases or 1.5 times the baseline
Acute haemorrhagic fever syndrome:	1 case
Acute jaundice syndrome:	5 cases or 1.5 times the baseline
Malaria:	5 cases or 1.5 times the baseline
Acute flaccid paralysis (suspected poliomyelitis):	1 case
Neonatal tetanus:	1 case
Fever of unknown origin:	1.5 times the baseline
Other communicable diseases:	1.5 times the baseline
Unknown disease occurring as a cluster:	report any cluster
Severe malnutrition:	2 cases

Baseline = average weekly number of cases of the disease calculated over the past 3 weeks.

---

1. SAMPLE WEEKLY MORBIDITY FORM

Province/Governorate: _____   District/Area: _____

Town/Village/Settlement/Camp: _____

Health facility: _____   Agency: _____

Reporting period: from Monday ____/____/_____   to Sunday ____/____/_____

Population covered: _____   Under-5 population: _____

Name of surveillance officer: _____

DISEASE / SYNDROME	NEW CASES	
	Under 5 years	5 years and over
* Acute watery diarrhoea		
* Bloody diarrhoea		
* Measles		
* Meningitis – suspected		
* Acute flaccid paralysis (suspected poliomyelitis)		
* Acute haemorrhagic fever syndrome		
* Acute jaundice syndrome		
^ Malaria – suspected		
Upper respiratory tract infection		
Acute lower respiratory tract infection/pneumonia		
Neonatal tetanus		
Fever of unknown origin		
Other communicable diseases		
* Unknown disease occurring as a cluster		

Trauma/injury:		
Landmine / UXO** injury		
War-related other than mine/UXO**		
Road traffic accident		
Other		
Severe malnutrition		
Mental health/stress-related problems		
Other non-communicable diseases		
TOTAL CLINIC ATTENDANCE		

* Diseases with outbreak potential – report as soon as possible to your health coordinator using outbreak alert form. See alert thresholds under "guidelines for use of surveillance forms".

** Unexploded ordnance

2. WEEKLY/MONTHLY DEMOGRAPHY FORM

Province/Governorate: _____   District/Area: _____

Town/Village/Settlement/Camp: _____

Health facility: _____   Agency: _____

Reporting period: from Monday _____/_____/_____   to Sunday _____/_____/_____

Name of surveillance officer: _____

	Children under 5 years (a)	Children over 5 years (b)	Total population (a + b)
Population at the end of last week/month (1)			
Births this week/month (2)			
Arrivals this week/month (3)			
Deaths this week/month (4)			
Departures this week/month (5)			
End of week/month population = (1 + 2 + 3 − 4 − 5)			

3. WEEKLY MORTALITY FORM

Province/Governorate: _____ District/Area: _____ Town/Village/Settlement/Camp: _____

Health facility (hospital/health centre): _____ Reporting period: from *Monday* ___/___/___ to Sunday ___/___/___

Population at the end of the week: _____ Under 5 population at the end of the week: _____

Name of surveillance officer: _____

No.	First and middle names	Family name	Sex (M/F)	Age (month/ years)	Direct causes of death														Underlying causes of death					Date of death (dd/mm/yy)	Location of death HF = health facility C = community	Lab. S = sample taken C = confirmed
					Acute watery diarrhoea *	Bloody diarrhoea	Measles	Meningitis (suspected)	Acute haemorrhagic fever syndrome	Acute jaundice syndrome	Malaria	ALRI/pneumonia	Trauma/injury *	Others *	Specify cause if known	Unknown	Neonatal death	Maternal death	Malnutrition	HIV/AIDS	Other (specify)			
1																									
2																									
3																									
4																									
5																									
6																									
7																									
8																									
9																									
10																									

§ See case definitions list.
* If this box is ticked, **also** specify cause in the "*specify cause*" column. Example: if cholera is suspected as the cause of the acute watery diarrhoea death, tick the acute watery diarrhoea column **and** write "cholera" in "*specify cause*" column. For **Trauma/injury** deaths: "*specify cause*" column should indicate 1 = mine/ UXO, 2 = war-related other than mine/UXO, 3 = RTA (road traffic accident), or 4 = other

5. Case definitions

✔ ACUTE WATERY DIARRHOEA

Three or more abnormally loose or fluid stools in the past 24 hours with or without dehydration.

To suspect case of cholera:

Person aged over 5 years with severe dehydration or death from acute watery diarrhoea with or without vomiting.

Person aged over 2 years with acute watery diarrhoea *in an area where there is a cholera outbreak.*

To confirm case of cholera:

Isolation of *Vibrio cholera* O1 or O139 from diarrhoeal stool sample.

✔ ACUTE HAEMORRHAGIC FEVER SYNDROME

Acute onset of fever of less than 3 weeks' duration in a severely ill patient **and** any two of the following:

- haemorrhagic or purpuric rash,
- epistaxis,
- haematemesis,
- haemoptysis,
- blood in stools,
- other haemorrhagic symptom and no known predisposing host factors for haemorrhagic manifestations.

✔ ACUTE JAUNDICE SYNDROME

Acute onset of jaundice **and** severe illness **and** absence of any known precipitating factors.

✔ ACUTE LOWER RESPIRATORY TRACT INFECTION/PNEUMONIA IN CHILDREN <5 YEARS

Cough or difficult breathing;

    and

Breathing 50 or more times per minute for infants aged 2 months to 1 year;

Breathing 40 or more times per minute for children aged 1 to 5 years;

    and

No chest indrawing, no stridor, no general danger signs.

Note: **Severe pneumonia** = Cough or difficult breathing **+** any general danger sign (unable to drink or breastfeed, vomits everything, convulsions, lethargic or unconscious) or chest indrawing or stridor in a calm child.

✔ ACUTE FLACCID PARALYSIS (SUSPECTED POLIOMYELITIS)

Acute flaccid paralysis in a child aged < 15 years, including Guillain-Barré syndrome **or** any paralytic illness in a person of any age.

To confirm case:

Laboratory-confirmed wild poliovirus in stool sample.

✔ BLOODY DIARRHOEA

Acute diarrhoea with visible blood in the stool.

To confirm case of epidemic bacillary dysentery:

Take stool specimen for culture and blood for serology. Isolation of *Shigella dysenteriae.*

✔ MALARIA – SUSPECTED

• *Uncomplicated malaria*

Patient with fever or history of fever within the past 48 hours (with or without other symptoms such as nausea, vomiting and diarrhoea, headache, back pain, chills, myalgia) in whom other obvious causes of fever have been excluded.

• *Severe malaria*

Patient with symptoms as for uncomplicated malaria, as well as drowsiness with extreme weakness and associated signs and symptoms related to organ failure such as disorientation, loss of consciousness, convulsions, severe anaemia, jaundice, haemoglobinuria, spontaneous bleeding, pulmonary oedema and shock.

To confirm case:

Demonstration of malaria parasites in blood film by examining thick or thin smears, or by rapid diagnostic test kit for *Plasmodium falciparum.*

✔ MEASLES

Fever **and** maculopapular rash (i.e. non-vesicular) **and** cough, coryza (i.e. runny nose) or conjunctivitis (i.e. red eyes);

or

Any person in whom a clinical health worker suspects measles infection.

To confirm case:

At least a fourfold increase in antibody titre **or** isolation of measles virus **or** presence of measles-specific IgM antibodies.

✔ MENINGITIS – SUSPECTED

Sudden onset of fever (> 38.0 °C axillary) **and** one of the following:
* neck stiffness,
* altered consciousness,
* other meningeal sign **or** petechial/purpural rash.

In children <1 year meningitis is suspected when fever is accompanied by a bulging fontanelle.

To confirm case:

Positive cerebrospinal fluid antigen detection **or** positive cerebrospinal fluid culture **or** positive blood culture.

✔ NEONATAL TETANUS

Suspected case:

Any neonatal death between 3 and 28 days of age in which the cause of death is unknown **or** any neonate reported as having suffered from neonatal tetanus between 3 and 28 days of age and not investigated.

To confirm case:

Any neonate with normal ability to suck and cry during the first 2 days of life, and who between 3 and 28 days of age cannot suck normally and becomes stiff or has convulsions (i.e. jerking of the muscles) or both.

Hospital-reported cases are considered confirmed.

The diagnosis is entirely clinical and does not depend on bacteriological confirmation.

✔ OTHER COMMUNICABLE DISEASES

These include some other communicable diseases not line-listed on the surveillance forms. The list below is non-exhaustive and details two outbreak-prone diseases in this category.

* *LEISHMANIASIS*

  – *Visceral leishmaniasis (VL)*

  Person with clinical signs of prolonged (>2 weeks) irregular fever, splenomegaly and weight loss, with serological (at peripheral geographical level) and/or (when feasible at central level) parasitological confirmation of the diagnosis.

  Note: In endemic malarious areas, visceral leishmaniasis must be suspected when fever not responding to anti-malarial drugs persists for more than 2 weeks (assuming drug-resistant malaria has also been considered).

  To confirm case:

  Positive parasitology

  – stained smears from bone marrow, spleen, liver, lymph node, blood

or

– culture of the organism from a biopsy or aspirated material

Positive serology (immunofluorescent assay, ELISA, Direct Agglutination Test)

– *Cutaneous leishmaniasis (CL)*

Person with clinical signs and parasitological confirmation of the diagnosis.

Clinical signs: Appearance of one or more skin lesions, typically on uncovered parts of the body. The face, neck, arms and legs are most common sites. A nodule may appear at the site of inoculation and may enlarge to become an indolent ulcer. The sore may remain in this stage for a variable time before healing – it typically leaves a depressed scar.

To confirm case:

Positive parasitology (stained smear or culture from the lesion).

• *TYPHOID FEVER*

Person with fever of at least 38 °C for 3 or more days is considered suspect if the epidemiological context is conducive.

Clinical diagnosis is difficult as it may vary from a mild illness with low grade fever and malaise to a severe picture of sustained fever, diarrhoea or constipation, anorexia, severe headache and intestinal perforation may occur.

To confirm case:

Isolation of *S.* Typhi from blood or stool cultures.

✔ **FEVER OF UNKNOWN ORIGIN**

Person with fever in whom all obvious causes of fever have been excluded.

✔ **UNKNOWN DISEASE OCCURRING AS A CLUSTER**

An aggregation of cases with related symptoms and signs of unknown cause that are closely grouped in time and/or place.

✔ **SEXUALLY TRANSMITTED DISEASES**

• *GENITAL ULCER SYNDROME*

Ulcer on penis or scrotum in men and on labia, vagina or cervix in women with or without inguinal adenopathy.

• *URETHRAL DISCHARGE SYNDROME*

Urethral discharge in men with or without dysuria.

- *VAGINAL DISCHARGE SYNDROME*

  Abnormal vaginal discharge (amount, colour and odour) with or without lower abdominal pain or specific symptoms or specific risk factors.

- *LOWER ABDOMINAL PAIN*

  Symptoms of lower abdominal pain and pain during sexual relations, with examination showing vaginal discharge, lower abdominal tenderness on palpation or temperature >38 °C.

✔ **SUSPECTED PULMONARY TUBERCULOSIS**

Any person who presents with symptoms or signs suggestive of pulmonary tuberculosis, in particular cough of long duration. May also have haemoptysis, chest pain, breathlessness, fever/night sweats, tiredness, loss of appetite and significant weight loss.

All TB suspects should have three sputum samples examined by light microscopy; early morning samples are more likely to contain the tuberculosis organism than a sample later in the day.

- *SMEAR-POSITIVE PULMONARY TUBERCULOSIS (PTB+)*

  Diagnostic criteria should include at least two sputum smear specimens positive for acid-fast bacilli (AFB);

  or

  One sputum smear specimen positive for AFB and radiographic abnormalities consistent with active pulmonary tuberculosis;

  or

  One sputum smear specimen positive for AFB and a culture positive for *M. tuberculosis.*

- *SMEAR-NEGATIVE PULMONARY TUBERCULOSIS (PTB–)*

  A case of pulmonary tuberculosis that does not meet the above definition for smear-positive tuberculosis. Diagnostic criteria should include at least three sputum smear specimens negative for AFB;

  and

  Radiographic abnormalities consistent with active pulmonary tuberculosis;

  and

  No response to a course of broad-spectrum antimicrobial;

  and

  Decision by a clinician to treat with a full course of antituberculosis chemotherapy.

✔ **MALNUTRITION**

Severe malnutrition:

In children 6 to 59 months (65 to 110 cm in height):

– weight-for-height (W/H) index < -3 Z scores (on table of NCHS/WHO normalized reference values of weight-for-height by sex);

– bilateral pitting oedema irrespective of W/H, in absence of other causes.

✔ TRAUMA/ INJURY

Injury (intentional)

A bodily lesion at the organic level, resulting from an intentionally inflicted acute exposure to energy in amounts that exceed the threshold of physiological tolerance.

Injury (non-intentional)

A bodily lesion at the organic level, resulting from a non-intentionally (i.e. "accidentally") inflicted acute exposure to energy in amounts that exceed the threshold of physiological tolerance.

Landmine/UXO injury

A person who has sustained, either directly or indirectly, a fatal or non-fatal injury caused by the explosion of a landmine or other unexploded ordnance (UXO).

Note: Landmine injuries relate to buried mines (e.g. antipersonnel and/or antivehicle mines).

UXO injuries arise from explosive objects/devices that are typically above ground at time of detonation, such as cluster munitions that did not detonate on impact.

Examples of other categories of trauma/injury that may be used for surveillance:

Trauma/injury other than landmine/UXO injury

Road traffic accident

Other

✔ MATERNAL DEATH

Death of a woman while pregnant or within 42 days of termination of pregnancy, regardless of the site or duration of pregnancy, from any cause related to or aggravated by the pregnancy or its management.

✔ NEONATAL DEATH

Death of a live-born infant in its first 28 days of life.

It is a classification by age not cause.

6. Outbreak investigation kit

SAMPLE OUTBREAK ALERT FORM

Province/Governorate: _____   District/Area: _____

Town/Village/Settlement/Camp: _____

Health facility: _____   Agency: _____

Date: _____/_____/_____

Name of reporting officer: _____

Symptoms and signs: you can tick several boxes	Suspected disease/syndrome: tick ONE box only
❑ Acute watery diarrhoea ❑ Bloody diarrhoea ❑ Fever ❑ Rash ❑ Cough ❑ Vomiting ❑ Neck stiffness ❑ Jaundice ❑ Bleeding ❑ Acute paralysis or weakness ❑ Increased secretions (e.g. sweating, drooling) ❑ Other: _____ **Total number of cases reported:**	❑ Acute watery diarrhoea ❑ Bacillary dysentery/shigellosis ❑ Cholera ❑ Measles ❑ Meningitis ❑ Malaria ❑ Acute flaccid paralysis (suspected poliomyelitis) ❑ Acute haemorrhagic fever syndrome ❑ Acute jaundice syndrome ❑ Cutaneous leishmaniasis ❑ Visceral leishmaniasis ❑ Typhoid fever ❑ Unknown disease occurring in a cluster ❑ Other: _____

Serial No.	Age	Sex	Location	Date of onset	Laboratory specimen taken (yes/no)	Treatment given	Outcome [a]	Final classi-fication [b]

[a] Outcome: I = currently ill; R = recovering or recovered; D = died.

[b] Final classification: S = suspected case with clinical diagnosis; C = confirmed case with laboratory diagnosis.

SAMPLE CASE INVESTIGATION FORM

Province/Governorate: _____   District/Area: _____

Town/Village/Settlement/Camp: _____

Health facility: _____   Agency: _____

Date: _____/_____/_____

Name of reporting officer: _____

1. PATIENT IDENTIFICATION

Case No.: _____   Name: _____

Location: _____

Date of birth: _____/_____/_____   Age: _____   Sex: **M**   **F**

2. CLINICAL DATA

Date of onset of illness: _____/_____/_____

- ❏ Acute watery diarrhoea
- ❏ Bloody diarrhoea
- ❏ Fever
- ❏ Rash
- ❏ Cough
- ❏ Vomiting
- ❏ Neck stiffness
- ❏ Jaundice
- ❏ Bleeding
- ❏ Acute paralysis or weakness
- ❏ Increased secretions (e.g. sweating, drooling)
- ❏ Other: _____

3. LABORATORY DATA

Sample: _____ Date taken: _____/_____/_____ Lab. received: _____/_____/_____

Name of laboratory: _____

Type of test: _____ Date of results: _____/_____/_____ Result: **Pos.** **Neg.**

4. FINAL CLASSIFICATION

Confirmed: Laboratory   Date of final diagnosis: _____/_____/_____

                    Clinical case

                                        Discarded final diagnosis: _____

5. FIELD INVESTIGATOR

Name: _____

Position: _____   Signature: _____

NOTE: ONE FORM PER CASE INVESTIGATED

OUTBREAK INVESTIGATION KIT

Item	Unit	Quantity/kit
1. Basic consumables module		
1.1 Cotton wool, BP, 100%, surgical quality	roll of 500 g	
1.2 Ballpoint pen		5
1.3 Pencil		5
1.4 Eraser		5
1.5 Felt-tip pen (waterproof)		5
1.6 Marking pen, water-resistant ink, black and blue		5
1.7 Notebook (A4, hard cover, squared paper)		5
1.8 Labels (blank, self-adhesive)	series	5
1.9 Ruler		5
1.10 Calculator		5
1.11 Scissors		5
1.12 Thermometer (0 −100°)		5
1.13 Torch (+ D-type spare batteries)		5
1.14 Sealing tape	roll	5
1.15 Normal saline (0.9%)	500 ml	5
1.16 Sharps container for disposal of needles and syringes, min. 2 litres		5
1.17 Chlorine granules 500 mg/containers		5
2. Common consumables for collection of all specimens		
2.1 Gauze swabs, 10 x 10 cm, 100% cotton, 12-ply, 17-thr, sterile	10 x 10 pcs/box	5
2.2 Disinfecting swabs, impregnated with 70% isopropyl alcohol	100/box	5
2.3 Microscope slides, 76 x 26 mm, cut edges	50/box	5
2.4 Cover glasses, 22 x 22 mm	1000/box	5
2.5 Storing box for microslides, wooden frame, for 25 pieces each	10/pack	5
2.6 Universal container, 70 ml, 55 x 44 mm, reliable sealing and PE cap, machine-sterile with standard label	1000/pack	5
2.7 Braunoderm (alcohol + PVP-IOD) for surgical scrub, against bacteria, fungi, viruses including HBV and HIV)	1 litre/contain	5
2.8 Povidone iodine solution	500 ml/contain	5
2.9 Alcoholic hand rub (+ pump dispenser)		5
3. Blood module		
3.1 Blood lancets, sterile, disposable	pack of 200	5
3.2 Monovettes (orange cap, 10 ml)	pack of 100	1
3.3 Monovettes (red cap, EDTA, 3 ml)	pack of 100	1
3.4 Needles for Monovettes 21G	pack of 100	1
3.5 Needles for Monovettes 23G	pack of 100	1
3.6 Butterfly needles for blood culture 21G	pack of 100	1
3.7 Disposable soft transfer pipettes	pack of 1000	1
3.8 Racks for blood tubes		5
3.9 Band aids (small)	pack	5
3.10 Blood culture bottles (Hemoline performance DUO, children)	12 vials/pack	5
3.11 Blood culture bottles (Hemoline performance diphasic)	12 vials/pack	5
3.12 Tourniquets with clip		5

Item	Unit	Quantity/kit
4. Respiratory module		
4.1 Tongue depressor	100/pack	5
4.2 Flexible wire calcium alginate tipped swab (for pertussis)	100/pack	1
4.3 Syringe for suction, 50/60 ml with catheter tip	60/pack	2
4.4 Transport swabs with Trans Amies transport medium	1000/pack	1
4.5 Virus transport medium (Cellmatics)	50/pack	1
5. Urine module		
5.1 Urine container with boric acid, PS w/screw cap, 30 ml (sterile)	400/pack	1
6. Stool module		
6.1 Rectal swabs for adults		25
6.2 Rectal swabs for infants		25
6.3 Stool collection tubes with spoon	400/pack	1
6.4 Tubes with Cary-Blair transport medium		100
7. CSF module		
7.1 Sterile cotton swab	100/pack	5
7.2 Bottle with Trans Isolate media		100
7.3 Spinal needle, 25G x 3.5	25/box	5
7.4 Spinal needles, 23G x 3.5	25/box	5
7.5 Needle for transfer into medium, 21G	?/box	
7.6 Microtube 2.0 ml, PP, with mouth screw cap and skirted base	50/bag	
7.7 Local anaesthetics (lidocaine 2% 2ml), 25G needle, 5-ml syringe		100
8. Self-protection module		
8.1 Disposable surgical gowns		10
8.2 Disposable surgical face masks	50 pcs/box	5
8.3 Disposable gloves: sizes S, M, L	100 pcs/box	5
8.4 Goggles		10
8.5 Face-mask type FFP3SL 3M brand		10
8.6 Disposable surgical caps, size M	50 pcs/box	5
8.7 Rubber surgical boots	pair, size 42	5
8.8 Disposable impermeable shoe cover, length 38 cm	100 pcs/bag	5
8.9 Impermeable aprons, 90 x 112 cm		5
8.10 Visors/face-shield		5
9. Specimen transport module		
9.1 Specimen carrier (cool box)		5
9.2 Icepacks	set of 24	5
9.3 Microcentrifuge tube rack		5
9.4 Complete combination packaging for infectious substances, BIOPACK 2 with 1.5-litre BIOJAR		5
9.5 CL-4 thermal control unit, polystyrene box set in fibreboard case with all labels and instructions		5

7. Organization of an isolation centre and calculation of treatment supplies

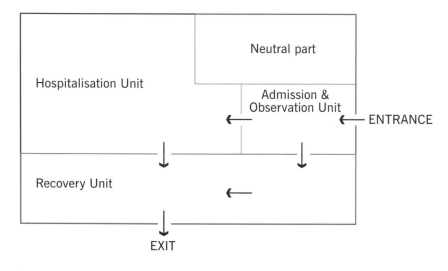

Four separate spaces:

• Admission and observation unit

• Neutral part: staff office and staff rest room, hospital kitchen, store rooms

• Hospitalisation unit: reserved for severe patients with IV fluids

• Recovery unit: oral rehydration space

In each space, ensure exclusive latrines, washing areas, large quantities of water and safe disposal of waste

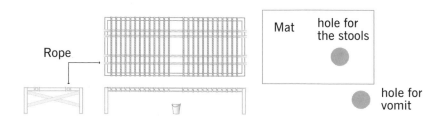

Figure A7.1   **Organization of an emergency treatment centre and patient-flow**

Table A7.1 **Essential rules in cholera treatment centre**

Mode of transmission	Essential rules in the CTC	Additional recommended rules
People	• Access limited to patient + one family member + staff • One-way flow of people	• Ideally one carer per patient only • 3 separate spaces within the centre (see box 1)
Water	• Safe water (chlorination concentration according to specific use; see Table A7.2) • Large quantity needed (minimum 10 litres/person/day)	• Ideally 50 litres per patient and per day
Hands	• Hand-washing stations with safe water and soap in sufficient quantities • Wash hands with water and soap • before and after taking care of patients • after going to the latrines • before cooking or eating after leaving the admission ward	• Cut and clean nails
Food	• Cooked food • Health care workers should not handle food or water	• Food provided by the CTC (preferably not by families) • Large stocks of food may be "tempting" and may lead to security problems
Clothes	• Wash clothes and linen with the appropriate chlorine solution	• If no chlorine available, wash clothes with soap and dry them in the sun
Environmental contamination (faeces and waste)	• Ensure exclusive latrines for the unit • Disinfect buckets, soiled surfaces and latrines regularly with the appropriate chlorine solution (see Table A7.2) • Incinerator for medical waste	• Latrines at least 100 metres away from wells or surface sources • Special cholera beds
Corpses	• Separate morgue • Disinfect corpses (see Table A7.2)	• Safe funeral practices • Dispose of corpses as soon as possible

Table A7.2 **Preparation and use of disinfectants**

Starting with:	2% SOLUTION	0.2% SOLUTION	0.05% SOLUTION
Calcium hypochlorite at 70% active chlorine ("high-test hypochlorite", "HTH")	30 g/litre or 2 tablespoons/litre	30 g/10 litres or 2 tablespoons/10 litres	7 g/10 litres or 1/2 tablespoon/10 litres
Chlorinated lime at 30% active chlorine ("bleaching powder")	66 g/litre or 4 tablespoons/litre	66 g/10 litres or 4 tablespoons/10 litres	16 g/10 litres or 1 tablespoon/10litres
Sodium hypochlorite solution at 6% active chlorine ("household bleach")	333 ml/litre or 22 tablespoons/litre	333 ml/10 litres or 22 tablespoons/10 litres	83 ml/10 litres or 5 tablespoons/10 litres
USE FOR DISINFECTION OF	Excreta Corpses Shoes	Floor Utensils Beds	Hands Skin Clothes

Measurements used: 1 teaspoon = 5 ml; 1 tablespoon = 15 ml; 1 cup = 200 ml.

Do not use metallic bucket for preparation and storage of chlorinated solutions

Table A7.3 **Cholera treatment supplies for an outbreak**

How to estimate the initial amount of supplies needed for a cholera outbreak
(0.2% of the population expected to fall ill initially)

The table below gives you an estimate of the amount of supplies you will need according to the number of people in your area. To find the amounts needed for each item, look in the column under the approximate population of your catchment area to the nearest 5000. You may add several columns (e.g. if your health facility serves 35 000 people, add the amounts in the 10 000 and 5000 columns to those in the 20 000 column). Write the amount needed at your health facility in the empty column on the right.

ITEM	**Population** (+ *numbers expected to fall ill*)						Your area
	5 000	10 000	15 000	20 000	50 000	100 000	
	(10)	(20)	(30)	(40)	(100)	(200)	
Rehydration supplies							
ORS packets (for 1 litre each)	65	130	195	260	650	1 300	
Nasogastric tubes (adults) 5.3/3.5 mm (16 Flack) 50 cm	1	1	1	2	3	6	
Nasogastric tubes (children)	1	1	1	2	3	6	
Ringer's lactate bags, 1 litre, with giving sets	12	24	36	48	120	240	
Scalp vein sets	2	3	4	5	10	20	
Antimicrobial							
Doxycycline, 100 mg (adults)	6	12	18	24	60	120	
Erythromycin, 250 mg (children)	24	48	72	96	240	480	
Other treatment supplies							
Large water dispensers with tap (marked at 5–10 litres)	1	1	1	2	2	4	
1-litre bottles for ORS solution	2	4	6	12	20	40	
0.5-litre bottles for ORS solution	2	4	6	12	20	20	
Tumblers, 200 ml	4	8	12	16	40	80	
Teaspoons	2	4	6	8	20	40	
Cotton wool, kg	1/2	1	1 1/2	2	5	10	
Adhesive tape, reels	1	1	1	2	3	6	

Developed by WHO Global Task Force on Cholera Control

Table A7.4　Dysentery treatment supplies per population

How to estimate the amount of supplies needed for a dysentery outbreak

(0.2% of the population expected to fall ill initially)

The table below gives you an estimate of the amount of supplies you will need according to the number of people in your area. To find the amounts needed for each item, look in the column under the approximate population of your catchment area to the nearest 5000. You may add several columns (e.g. if your health facility serves 35 000 people, add the amounts in the 10 000 and 5000 columns to those in the 20 000 column). Write the amount needed at your health facility in the empty column on the right.

	Population (+ *numbers expected to fall ill*)						Your area
	5 000	10 000	15 000	20 000	50 000	100 000	
ITEM	(10)	(20)	(30)	(40)	(100)	(200)	
Rehydration supplies							
ORS packets (for 1 litre each)	10	20	30	40	100	200	
Ringer's lactate bags, 1 litre, with giving sets	2	4	6	8	20	40	
Scalp vein sets	1	1	2	2	5	10	
Antimicrobial							
Ciprofloxacin, 500 mg	100	200	300	400	1000	2000	
Other treatment supplies							
Large water dispensers with tap (marked at 5–10 litres)	1	1	1	1	1	2	
1-litre bottles for ORS solution	1	1	2	2	5	10	
0.5-litre bottles for ORS solution	1	1	2	2	5	10	
Tumblers, 200 ml	1	2	3	4	10	20	
Teaspoons	1	1	2	2	5	10	
Cotton wool, kg	1/2	1	11/2	2	5	10	
Adhesive tape, reels	1	1	1	2	3	6	
Hand soap, kg	2	4	6	8	20	40	
Boxes of soap for washing clothes	3	6	9	12	30	60	
1-litre bottle of cleaning solution (2% chlorine or 1–2% phenol)	1	1	1	1	2	4	

Developed by WHO Global Task Force on Cholera Control

Table A7.5   **Typhoid fever treatment supplies per population**

How to estimate the amount of supplies needed for a typhoid outbreak
(0.2% of the population expected to fall ill initially)

The table below gives you an estimate of the amount of supplies you will need according to the number of people in your area. To find the amounts needed for each item, look in the column under the approximate population of your catchment area to the nearest 5000. You may add several columns (e.g. if your health facility serves 35 000 people, add the amounts in the 10 000 and 5000 columns to those in the 20 000 column). Write the amount needed at your health facility in the empty column on the right. On the basis of drug resistance in your area, choose only one of the antimicrobial.

ITEM	Population (+ *numbers expected to fall ill*)						Your area
	5 000	10 000	15 000	20 000	50 000	100 000	
	(10)	(20)	(30)	(40)	(100)	(200)	
Rehydration supplies							
ORS packets (for 1 litre each)	10	20	30	40	100	200	
Ringer's lactate bags* 1 litre, with giving sets	1	2	3	4	10	20	
Scalp vein sets	1	1	2	2	5	10	
Antimicrobial							
Chloramphenicol, 250 mg	2500	5000	7500	10000	25000	50000	
Amoxicillin, 500 mg	1680	3360	5040	6720	16800	33600	
Co-trimoxazole, (SMX 400 mg + TMP 80 mg)	840	1680	2520	3360	8400	16800	
Cefixime, 200mg **	840	1680	2520	3360	8400	16800	
Other treatment supplies							
Large water dispensers with tap (marked at 5–10 litres)	1	1	1	1	1	2	
1-litre bottles for ORS solution	1	1	2	2	5	10	
0.5-litre bottles for ORS solution	1	1	2	2	5	10	
Tumblers, 200 ml	1	2	3	4	10	20	
Teaspoons	1	1	2	2	5	10	
Cotton wool, kg	1/2	1	1 1/2	2	5	10	
Adhesive tape, reels	1	1	1	2	3	6	
Hand soap, kg	2	4	6	8	20	40	
Box of soap for washing clothes	3	6	9	12	30	60	
1-litre bottle of cleaning solution (2% chlorine or 1–2% phenol)	1	1	1	1	2	4	

Considering that less than 50% of the patients need IV rehydration.
** *In case of multidrug resistance to above antimicrobial, choose Cefixime.*
Developed by WHO Global Task Force on Cholera Control

8. Collection of specimens for laboratory analysis

A8.1 BLOOD SPECIMEN COLLECTION

Blood and separated serum are the most common specimens taken in outbreaks of communicable disease. Venous blood can be used for direct isolation of the pathogen, or separated into serum for the detection of genetic material (e.g. by polymerase chain reaction), specific antibodies (by serology), antigens or toxins (e.g. by immunofluorescence). Serum is preferable to unseparated blood for the processing of most specimens for diagnosis of viral pathogens, except where otherwise directed. When specific antibodies are being assayed, it is often helpful to collect paired sera, i.e. an acute sample at the onset of illness and a convalescent sample 1–4 weeks later. Blood can also collected by finger prick for the preparation of slides for microscopy or for absorption on to special filter paper discs for analysis. Whenever possible, blood specimens for culture should be taken before antimicrobial are administered to the patient.

Materials for collection of venous blood samples

- Skin disinfection: 70% alcohol (isopropanol) or 10% povidone iodine, swabs, gauze pads, band-aids.
- Disposable latex or vinyl gloves.
- Tourniquet, Vacutainer® or similar vacuum blood collection devices, or disposable syringes and needles.
- Sterile screw-cap tubes (or cryotubes if indicated), blood culture bottles (50 ml for adults, 25 ml for children) with appropriate media.
- Labels and indelible marker pen.

Method of collection

- Place a tourniquet above the venepuncture site. Disinfect the tops of blood culture bottles.
- Palpate and locate the vein. It is critical to disinfect the venepuncture site meticulously with 10% polyvidone iodine or 70% isopropanol by swabbing the skin concentrically from the centre of the venepuncture site outwards. Let the disinfectant evaporate. Do not repalpate the vein. Perform venepuncture.
- If withdrawing with conventional disposable syringes, withdraw 5–10 ml of whole blood from adults, 2–5 ml from children and 0.5–2 ml from infants. Under asepsis, transfer the specimen to appropriate transport tubes and culture bottles. Secure caps tightly.

- If withdrawing with vacuum systems, withdraw the desired amount of blood directly into each transport tube and culture bottle.
- Remove the tourniquet. Apply pressure to site until bleeding stops and apply adhesive dressing.
- Label the tubes, including the unique patient identification number, using an indelible marker pen.
- Do not recap used sharps. Discard directly into the sharps disposal container.
- Complete the case investigation and the laboratory request forms using the same identification number.

Handling and transport

Blood specimen bottles and tubes should be transported upright and secured in a screw cap container or in a rack in a transport box. They should have enough absorbent paper around them to soak up all the liquid in case of spillage.

If the specimen will reach the laboratory within 24 hours, most pathogens can be recovered from blood cultures transported at ambient temperature. Keep at 4–8 °C for longer transit periods, unless a cold-sensitive bacterial pathogen is suspected such as meningococcus, pneumococcus, *Shigella* spp.

A8.2 BLOOD SPECIMEN COLLECTION FOR VHF INVESTIGATION

All invasive procedures and investigations should be minimized until the diagnosis of VHF is confirmed or excluded. Only the specific diagnostic samples needed should be obtained from acutely ill patients. Other routine blood samples should be avoided when investigating a case of viral haemorrhagic fever.

The blood samples should be kept in their original tube (sealed sterile dry tubes, Monovettes or Vacutainer® type).

Do **not** attempt to separate serum or plasma from blood clots in the field, this may be highly risky in case of VHFs. These procedures should be performed at the reference laboratory.

Each collected sample must be identified as "High risk", and labels prepared in advance for both specimens collected including laboratory request forms. Labels should include name, date of collection and a code for the link with the corresponding case record.

Precautions for sampling

When investigating cases of VHFs, strict basic safety precautions must be taken. Some additional specific precautions and safety equipment are required to protect skin and mucous membranes against these pathogens.

Blood specimens should be taken by a doctor or nurse experienced in the procedure. Urine samples also should be handled carefully; a 20-ml syringe may be used to transfer urine from a bedpan to the specified container.

Always wear protective clothing when handling specimens from suspected VHF cases:

- a protective gown,
- a waterproof protective apron,
- two pairs of latex gloves,
- particulate filter face mask,
- goggles,
- rubber boots.

Method of collection

- Observe all the basic safety precautions when obtaining specimens samples from suspected VHF cases.
- For taking blood samples, it is advisable the use of a vacuum blood sampling system (Monovette or Vacutainer®). However, you may use the most familiar equipment and procedure to avoid the risk of accidents or spills.
- Withdraw 5–10 ml of whole blood from adults, 2–5 ml from children and 0.5–2 ml from infants, directly in the transport tube (blood sample tube).
- Avoid the use of disposable alcohol swabs to apply pressure to venopucture wounds. It is advisable to use dry cotton wool balls or gauze swabs.
- After taking the sample, disinfect the blood sample tube externally by wiping with hypochlorite solution of 0.5% (see A8.7).

Taking off protective clothing

- When finished, remove the apron; before removing the outer pair of gloves, wash your hands with soap and water and rinse them in hypochlorite solution 0.5% (see A8.7) for one minute.
- Keep the inner gloves on while removing goggles, mask, anything used to cover the head,the external gown and boots (the boots should also have been previously soaked in same hypochlorite solution).
- Finally remove the gloves and the inner gown, wash your hands well with soap and water and disinfect them with 70% isopropanol or povidone iodine.
- Dispose of all protective clothing, gloves, and materials in a plastic bag and incinerate everything. Remember to never recap used sharps. Discard directly into sharps disposal container for later incineration.

Handling and transport

Special care must be taken to prevent external contamination of specimen containers during specimen collection.

Three package system:

- The blood sample tube should be transported upright and secured in a screw-cap, leak-proof secondary container with sufficient absorbent material to absorb all the contents should leakage occur. Be sure the cap is screwed tight and the tube labelled (specimen record). The secondary container should be externally disinfected by wiping with 0.5% hypochlorite solution 0.5% (see A8.7).
- Specimen data forms and information that identifies or describes the specimen and also identifies the shipper and receiver should be taped to the outside of the secondary receptacle.
- The secondary container is finally placed into a third container (transport box). The outer part of the transport box should be clearly and visibly labelled with the biohazard label and the address. It must also clearly identify the type of specimen, the shipper and the receiver.
- If the blood sample cannot be processed the same day, ice-packs must be placed into the transport box in order to keep the sample cold (around 4 °C– 8 °C).
- **Whole blood sample should not be frozen.**

A8.3 CEREBROSPINAL FLUID (CSF) SPECIMEN COLLECTION

The specimen must be taken by a physician or a person experienced in the procedure. CSF is used in the diagnosis of viral, bacterial, parasitic and fungal meningitis/encephalitis.

Materials for collection

A lumbar puncture tray should be used that includes:

- sterile materials: gloves, cotton wool, towels or drapes,
- local anaesthetic, needle, syringe,
- skin disinfectant: 10% polyvidone iodine or 70% isopropanol,
- two lumbar puncture needles, small bore with stylet,
- six small sterile screw-cap tubes and tube rack,
- water manometer (optional),
- microscope slides and slide boxes.

Method of collection

As only experienced personnel should be involved in the collection of CSF samples, the method is not described here. CSF is collected directly into the separate screw-cap tubes. If the sample is not to be promptly transported, separate samples should be collected for bacterial and viral processing.

Handling and transport

In general, specimens should be delivered to the laboratory and processed as soon as possible.

CSF specimens for bacteriology are transported at ambient temperature, generally without transport media. They must never be refrigerated, as these pathogens do not survive well at low temperatures.

CSF specimens for virology do not need a transport medium. They may be transported at 4–8 °C for up to 48 hours, or at –70 °C for longer periods.

Rapid diagnostic tests

Several commercial kits are available, based on the direct detection of *N. meningitidis* antigens in CSF by latex agglutination tests. Follow the manufacturer's instructions precisely when using these tests. For best results, test the supernatant of the centrifuged CSF sample as soon as possible. If immediate testing is not possible, the sample can be refrigerated (between 2 °C and 8 °C) for up to several hours, or frozen at –20 °C for longer periods. Reagents should be kept refrigerated between 2 °C and 8 °C when not in use. Product deterioration occurs at higher temperatures, especially in tropical climates, and test results may become unreliable before the expiry date of the kit. Latex suspensions should never be frozen. Note that some kits have a working temperature range and tropical temperatures may be above the recommended upper limit.

A8.4 FAECAL SPECIMEN COLLECTION

Stool specimens are most useful for microbiological diagnosis if collected soon after onset of diarrhoea (for viruses < 48 hours and for bacteria < 4 days) and preferably before the initiation of antimicrobial therapy. If required, two or three specimens may be collected on separate days. Stool is the preferred specimen for culture of bacterial and viral diarrhoeal pathogens. Rectal swabs from faeces of infants may also be used for bacterial culture, but they are not useful for the diagnosis of viruses and of little value for the diagnosis of parasites. See figure A8.1 for sampling and transport procedures for cholera and *Shigella* spp.

Materials for collection
- Clean, dry, leak, proof-screw cap container and adhesive tape.
- Appropriate bacterial transport media for transport of rectal swabs from infants.
- Parasitology transport pack: 10% formalin in water, polyvinyl isopropyl alcohol (PVA).

Method of collecting a stool specimen
- Collect freshly passed stool, 5 ml liquid or 5 g solid (pea-size), in a container.
- Label the container.

Method of collecting a rectal swab from infants

- Moisten a swab in sterile saline.
- Insert the swab tip just past the anal sphincter and rotate gently.
- Withdraw the swab and examine to ensure that the cotton tip is stained with faeces.
- Place the swab in a sterile tube/container containing the appropriate transport medium.
- If necessary, break off the top part of the stick without touching the inside of the tube and tighten the screw cap firmly.
- Label the specimen tube.

Handling and transport

Stool specimens should be transported at 4–8°C. Bacterial yields may fall significantly if specimens are not processed within 1–2 days of collection. *Shigella* spp. are particularly sensitive to elevated temperatures.

Cholera specimens do not need refrigeration. With Cary-Blair transport medium, the sample needs to reach the laboratory within 7 days. Without a transport medium, the specimen must be transported to the laboratory within 2 hours (a cotton-tipped rectal swab soaked in liquid stool placed in sterile tube or bag/filter paper soaked with liquid stool with 2 or 3 drops of normal saline NaCl 9% can be used.)

Specimens to be examined for parasites should be mixed with 10% formalin or PVA, three parts stool to one part preservative. They should be transported at ambient temperature in containers sealed in plastic bags.

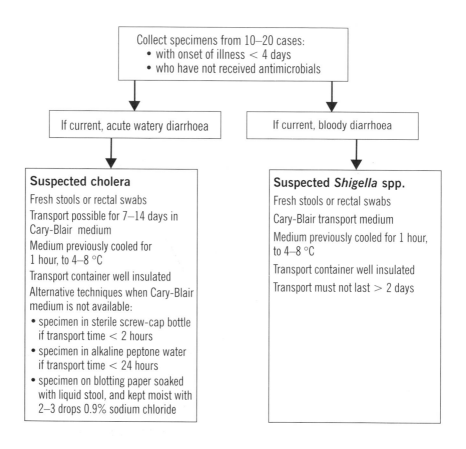

Figure A8.1 **Stool sampling and transport procedures for cholera and *Shigella* spp.**

A8.5 RESPIRATORY TRACT SPECIMEN COLLECTION

Specimens are collected from the upper or lower respiratory tract, depending on the site of infection. Upper respiratory tract pathogens (viral and bacterial) are found in throat and nasopharyngeal specimens. Lower respiratory tract pathogens are found in sputum specimens. For organisms such as *Legionella*, culture is difficult, and diagnosis is best based on the detection of antigen excreted in the urine.

When acute epiglottitis is suspected, no attempt should be made to take throat or pharyngeal specimens since these procedures may precipitate respiratory obstruction. Epiglottitis is generally confirmed by lateral neck X-ray, but the etiological agent may be isolated on blood culture.

Materials for collection

- Transport media – bacterial and viral.
- Dacron and cotton swabs.
- Tongue depressor.
- Flexible wire calcium alginate tipped swab (for suspected pertussis).
- Nasal speculum (for suspected pertussis – not essential).
- Suction apparatus or 20–50 ml syringe.
- Sterile screw-cap tubes and wide-mouthed clean sterile jars (minimum volume 25 ml).

UPPER RESPIRATORY TRACT SPECIMENS

Method of collecting a throat swab

- Hold the tongue down with the depressor. Use a strong light source to locate areas of inflammation and exudate in the posterior pharynx and the tonsillar region of the throat behind the uvula.
- Rub the area back and forth with a dacron or calcium alginate swab. Withdraw the swab without touching the cheeks, teeth or gums and insert into a screw-cap tube containing transport medium.
- If necessary, break off the top part of the stick without touching the inside of the tube and tighten the screw cap firmly.
- Label the specimen containers.
- Complete the laboratory request form.

Method of collecting nasopharyngeal swabs (for suspected pertussis)

- Seat the patient comfortably, tilt the head back and insert the nasal speculum.
- Insert a flexible calcium alginate/dacron swab through the speculum parallel to the floor of the nose without pointing upwards. Alternatively, bend the swab and insert it into the throat and move the swab upwards into the nasopharyngeal space.
- Rotate the swab on the nasopharyngeal membrane a few times, remove it carefully and insert it into a screw-cap tube containing transport medium.
- If necessary, break off the top part of the swab without touching the inside of the tube and tighten the screw cap firmly.
- Label the specimen tube.
- Complete the laboratory request form.

LOWER RESPIRATORY TRACT SPECIMENS

Method of collecting sputum

- Instruct the patient to take a deep breath and cough up sputum directly into a wide-mouth sterile container.

- Avoid saliva or postnasal discharge. The minimum volume should be about 1 ml. Label the specimen containers.
- Complete the laboratory request form.
- Always label the jar, NOT the lid.

Handling and transport

- All respiratory specimens, except sputum, are transported in appropriate bacterial/viral media.
- Transport as quickly as possible to the laboratory to reduce overgrowth by commensal oral flora.
- For transit periods up to 24 hours, transport bacterial specimens at ambient temperature and viruses at 4–8 °C in appropriate media.

A8.6 URINE SPECIMEN COLLECTION

Materials for collection

- Sterile plastic cup with lid (50 ml or more).
- Clean, screw-top specimen transport containers ("universal" containers are often used).
- Gauze pads.
- Soap and clean water (or normal saline) if possible.

Method of collection

- Give the patient clear instructions to pass urine for a few seconds, and then to hold the cup in the urine stream for a few seconds to catch a mid-stream urine sample. This should decrease the risk of contamination from organisms living in the urethra.
- To decrease the risk of contamination from skin organisms, the patient should be directed to avoid touching the inside or rim of the plastic cup with the skin of the hands, legs or external genitalia. Tighten the cap firmly when finished.
- For hospitalized or debilitated patients, it may be necessary to wash the external genitalia with soapy water to reduce the risk of contamination. If soap and clean water are not available, the area may be rinsed with normal saline. Dry the area thoroughly with gauze pads before collecting the urine.
- Urine collection bags may be necessary for infants. If used, transfer urine from the urine bag to specimen containers as soon as possible to prevent contamination with skin bacteria. Use a disposable transfer pipette to transfer the urine.
- Label the specimen containers.

Handling and transport

Transport to the laboratory within 2–3 hours of collection. If this is not possible, do not freeze but keep the specimen refrigerated at 4–8 °C to reduce the risk of overgrowth of contaminating organisms.

Cholera specimens do not need refrigeration. With Cary-Blair transport medium, the samples need to reach the laboratory within 7 days. Without a transport medium, the specimens must be transported to the laboratory within 2 hours (a cotton-tipped rectal swab soaked in liquid stool placed in sterile tube or bag; or filter paper soaked with liquid stool with 2 or 3 drops of normal saline NcCl 9% can be used).

Ensure that transport containers are leak-proof and tightly sealed.

A8.7 CHEMICAL DISINFECTANTS

Disinfection

Chlorine is the recommended disinfectant for use in field laboratories. An all-purpose disinfectant should have a working concentration of 0.1% (= 1 g/litre = 1000 ppm) of available chlorine. A stronger solution of 0.5% (= 5 g/litre = 5000 ppm) available chlorine should be used in situations such as suspected viral haemorrhagic fever outbreaks.

In preparing appropriate dilutions, remember that different products have different concentrations of available chlorine. To prepare solutions with the above concentrations, the manufacturer may provide appropriate instructions. Otherwise, use the guidelines provided below. Chlorine solutions gradually lose strength, and freshly diluted solutions must therefore be prepared daily. Clear water should be used because organic matter destroys chlorine.

Commonly used chlorine-based disinfectants include:

- sodium hypochlorite;
- commercial liquid bleaches such as household bleach (e.g. Chlorox®, Eau-de-Javel), which generally contain 5% (50 g/litre or 50 000 ppm) available chlorine.

However, the latter preparations lose a proportion of their chlorine content over time. Thick bleach solutions should never be used directly for disinfection purposes in disasters as they contain potentially poisonous additives.

To prepare a 0.1% chlorine solution with commercial bleach, make a 1 in 50 dilution, i.e. 1 part bleach in 49 parts water to give final concentrations of available chlorine of 0.1%. (For example, this could entail adding 20 ml of bleach to approximately 1 litre of water.)

Similarly, to make a 0.5% chlorine solution, make a 1 in 10 dilution, i.e. 1 part bleach in 9 parts water to give final concentrations of available chlorine of 0.5% (e.g. add 100 ml of bleach to 900 ml water.)

Chloramine powder

While the above-described bleach solution may satisfy all disinfection needs, chloramine powder may prove convenient for the disinfection of spills of blood and other potentially infectious body fluids. It may also prove useful under field conditions because of ease of transport. It contains approximately 25% available chlorine. In addition to its use as a powder on spills, chloramine powder may be used to prepare liquid chlorine solutions. The recommended formula is 20 g of chloramine powder to 1 litre of clean water.

Decontamination of surfaces

Wear an apron, heavy-duty gloves and other barrier protection if needed. Disinfect surfaces by wiping clean with 0.1% chlorine solution, then incinerate all absorbent material in heavy-duty garbage bags.

Decontamination of blood or body fluid spills

For spills, chloramine granules should be very liberally sprinkled to absorb the spill and left for at least 30 minutes. If chloramine powder is not available, one may use 0.5% chlorine solution to inactivate pathogens before soaking up the fluid with absorbent materials. These absorbent materials must then be incinerated.

Sterilization and reuse of instruments and materials

In field outbreak situations, it is not advisable to consider sterilization and reuse of any instruments or materials. Sterilization techniques are therefore not required and are not described here

Disinfection of hands

The principal means for disinfecting hands is by washing with soap and water. If available, one may also use commercial hand disinfectants containing chlorhexidine or polyvidone iodine.

9. Setting up a diagnostic laboratory

A diagnostic laboratory should comply with a number of essential principles.

- It must be able to undertake the types of test required.
- It must be able to handle the specimen load.
- It must be safe and comfortable for the staff to work in.
- If it is established in a community (rather than in a temporary camp) it should be sustainable in the long term.

To meet these needs the laboratory should have:

- A suitable building or room(s) appropriately laid out and furnished.
- Adequate numbers of staff who have been trained in the tests to be undertaken.
- Defined standard operating procedures covering the tests to be undertaken.
- Internal and external quality control to ensure consistency and accuracy of output.
- A safety policy based on the tests undertaken and the risks posed by the organisms present in the area.
- The appropriate equipment, reagents, media, glassware and disposables.
- Technical, engineering and logistic support.
- Good access and external communications.

Any departure from the most basic type of laboratory implies a marked increase in complexity and expense, and a concomitant increase in the difficulties of maintaining the unit and providing suitable staff.

LABORATORY PREMISES

Laboratories should provide an adequate level of secondary (environmental) containment to allow safe working within and to protect those using the area around the laboratory from microbiological risk. In acute emergencies, almost any accommodation that can provide cover from the sun and rain has at one time or another been used for laboratory work. While a tent or plastic sheeting can be so used, the ability of the staff to do useful work is likely to be rapidly degraded by poor working conditions and proper accommodation should be provided as soon as possible.

Any building or room that is to be used as a laboratory should be structurally sound. This includes the walls, roofs, floors, ceilings, doors and windows. The internal surfaces should be sealed with oil paint or varnish so that they can easily be cleaned or disinfected and to prevent dust falling onto work surfaces.

Windows should fit, be able to open, and be provided with security grilles and mosquito screens where appropriate. External doors should be lockable and not open directly into the laboratory but into a service corridor. Entrances to staff rooms, toilets, etc. should also be off this corridor. If only latrines are available they should be of the VIP type and reasonably close to the laboratory. Adequate hand-washing facilities must be provided at the exit to the laboratory room and for those using the toilet facilities/latrines. A specimen reception area should be provided that is outside the main laboratory suite and off the service corridor.

If the laboratory itself cannot be locked when it is empty, suitable security measures (e.g. lockable cupboards) must be taken to protect valuable equipment such as microscopes.

Benches

Laboratories must have good stable work surfaces. Ideally, these should be totally resistant to all likely disinfectants (hypochlorites, phenolics, aldehydes, alcohols and detergents), acids, alkalis and solvents. The best surfaces are special laminates that are resistant to chemical attack and heat, and sufficiently scratch-resistant (kitchen work surfaces are rarely adequate). However, in the basic laboratories used in emergencies it is more common to find wooden tables or benches in use. Polished surfaces do not resist chemicals and solvents well and may trap microorganisms. Any gaps in the table surface should be filled and levelled before the surface is varnished.

Benches should be of a suitable height (90 cm is commonly used). Consideration should also be given to the possible need to put small refrigerators, cupboards and drawer units under benches when bench heights are selected. Laboratory seating should be of adequate height to allow sustained comfortable working at the bench (stools of some type are ideal) and should also be able to be decontaminated without damage with the same range of disinfectants to be used on the benching.

Laboratory services

- A suitable building or room(s) appropriately laid out and furnished.
- Adequate water supplies are essential. The laboratory may need its own well. Water tanks should be covered to keep out dust and wildlife. If the supply is contaminated, some form of purification system (e.g. filtration and possibly chemical disinfection) may be needed. The laboratory will also need a still to provide pure, mineral-free water.
- Hand-washing facilities should be provided by the exit door of each laboratory.
- A glassware wash-up and drying area will be needed and this should ideally be in a separate room.

- Adequate drainage must be provided. Large soakaways may be required. If town drainage is used adequate trapping must be fitted to the laboratory waste system to allow for the trapping of any chemical or biological spills before they contaminate the town system.
- The laboratory should be provided with an incinerator.
- Complex autoclaves are generally not suitable for emergency laboratories. Autoclaving should usually be limited to the simple domestic pressure cooker or basic bench type.

Disposal of laboratory waste

- A suitable building or room(s) appropriately laid out and furnished.
- Liquid microbiological waste should be either heat-treated or chemically treated before discard into the drainage system. If chemical decontamination is used, any runoff from the drainage system must not be able to contaminate potable water sources.
- All solid waste containing infectious material or potentially infectious material should be incinerated.
- Disposal bins must be provided for sharps and the contents incinerated.

Electricity and gas

- Adequate electricity supplies are likely to be needed. The amount needed will depend on the number of items of equipment and whether they need to be run continuously.

  If local electricity supplies are intermittent or inadequate a generator may be needed. The capacity of the generator will be governed by the anticipated load and whether it is needed for continuous or occasional use. If all the laboratory electricity comes from its own generator and some of the laboratory equipment needs to run continuously, a backup generator is essential. If intermittent town supplies are used, an automatic system to switch on the generator if the town supplies fail may be needed. A battery reserve (with inverters) may be needed to cover gaps in the supply. Batteries may be kept charged by a solar system and the need for such a system (and its sustainability) should be investigated.
- Gas (propane/butane) may be required for Bunsen burners and/or gas refrigerators. This will depend on the availability of supplies of bottled gas and on the ability of engineering staff or local tradesmen to maintain such a system.

Environmental controls (ventilation, temperature, and humidity)

- Ventilation and airflow in basic laboratories (e.g. microscopy laboratories) are usually provided via the windows and doors. All windows should be fitted with a means of shading them from the sun. The ideal method is the use of external shutters hinged at the top and with a support stay. Doors may have a grille fitted near floor level to allow air entry.

- In laboratories where pathogens are routinely handled a predictable unidirectional airflow across and out of the laboratory should be maintained when the facility is in use so as to protect the workforce. This can be achieved by the use of extraction fans situated on one side of the laboratory, preferably the opposite side to opening windows and doors. Windows on the extractor fan side of the laboratory should not be capable of opening. Work with infectious risk should be conducted towards the extraction fan side of the room. Non-infectious work/record keeping should be done on the opening window/door side.

- When determining the layout of the laboratory account should be taken of:
  - the prevailing wind direction,
  - the situation of other buildings, paths, etc. and the use made of the space around the laboratory building.
  This is to ensure that the air from the laboratory is not vented into areas where people may be at risk from contaminants. Ducted air extraction may be needed.

- Any diagnostic laboratory should aim to work within certain defined temperature limits. It should be recognised that good laboratory practice (GLP) for the protection of workers (i.e. wearing of lab coats, gloves, masks for respiratory protection, eye protection) cannot be followed easily in extreme temperatures (>30 ºC) or high humidity. It should also be noted that many commercial diagnostic assays perform unpredictably, above 28–30 ºC and that equipment (especially refrigerators) usually works better when it is not too hot. Equally, satisfactory working becomes impossible when it is too cold. Control of temperature is extremely difficult in tented accommodation or in laboratories built from plastic sheeting which is one reason why such accommodation should be regarded as temporary.

- The control of temperature and humidity may require an air conditioned/cooled environment. Recirculating air conditioning is not suited to microbiological laboratories since this may recirculate and concentrate infectious risks to workers. Chiller systems are preferred but must be sited with regard for cross-laboratory airflow. Fans should generally be avoided as they can spread infectious material around and blow it into the faces of workers.

Vector/pest control

Insects, rodents and any other pests must be kept out of the laboratory area. Such pests may interfere with the work of the laboratory or contaminate media, etc. but in addition also risk the spread of pathogens from the laboratory to the outside thus compromising secondary containment. Windows should therefore be fitted with insect screens.

STAFF

In the early phases of a disaster only well trained staff should be employed for technical work. There will not be sufficient time to train laboratory assistants. The technical staff employed should be experienced in the relevant fields (particularly parasitology and haematology, although some knowledge of biochemistry, bacteriology and virology may be needed). At least one should have had experience of running a laboratory, preferably in field conditions, and be able to undertake additional duties such as laboratory management, ordering stock, etc.

As the situation stabilizes, the opportunity to increase the numbers of staff and to begin training or retraining local staff can begin.

TYPES OF TEST

In the acute emergency phase it is likely that only basic laboratory facilities can be established and hence only a limited number of tests can be offered. As the situation stabilizes it will be possible to establish a more sophisticated laboratory and hence to offer a wider range of tests.

1. Acute emergency phase

Microorganisms:

- malaria – microscopy and/or spot tests,
- meningococcal meningitis – spot tests,
- stool examinations for ova and parasites,
- detection of bloodborne agents other than malaria (trypanosomes, leishmanias, rickettsia),
- HIV and HepB (if blood transfusions are being given).

It is of value to have a means of culturing and identifying *Shigella dysenteriae* and *Vibrio cholerae* but this will rarely be possible in small basic laboratories. Links with nearby laboratories capable of offering this service should be considered.

Basic haematology:

- haematocrit (packed cell volume),
- differential white cell counts,
- sickle-cell detection,
- clotting time,
- typing and cross-matching blood (if blood transfusions are being undertaken).

2. Post-emergency phase

At this stage, tests for less acute conditions can be included. For example TB is a growing problem in many parts of the world and can spread readily in the crowded conditions often found in refugee and IDP camps. Sputum microscopy for the diagnosis of TB can easily be practised in basic conditions but it is worth doing only if the condition can be treated and this should only be done in the context of a properly designed and functioning DOTS programme.

STANDARD OPERATING PROCEDURES AND QUALITY CONTROL

Merely meeting the basic design and safety criteria for diagnostic laboratories is not enough. The staff must be able to undertake the required tests effectively and accurately. The output of the laboratory must be validated and a quality control system is essential. The way in which all diagnostic procedures undertaken in a laboratory should be performed should be laid down in "Standard Operating Procedures" (SOPs). These should include reference to full risk and hazard assessments and safety procedures. Protocols for internal and external quality assessment should also be laid down in these SOPs.

INTERNAL QUALITY CONTROL

All procedures undertaken in the laboratory must be measured against recognized standards. New batches of stains or reagents must be validated against the old. The work of the laboratory staff should be validated regularly by the blind inclusion of known positive and negative specimens in the routine diagnostic work.

EXTERNAL QUALITY CONTROL

A suitable body to undertake external quality control should be identified as soon as possible after the establishment of the laboratory. This agency should provide known positive and negative specimens for assessment of the work of the laboratory.

DISEASE RISKS

Any agency intending to undertake medical work in an area should obtain detailed information as to the spectrum of diseases that it will have to deal with. This is essential both for the design of the laboratory "package" required and will help determine the microbiological risks that may face its staff (all its staff, not just laboratory staff members). The risks posed by any organism likely to be encountered can be classified according to the following criteria:

- pathogenicity;
- mode of transmission and host range can be influenced by:
    - existing levels of immunityion,
    - host population movements,

- – vectors and reservoirs,
- – weather,
- – environmental factors (topography, plant species and distribution, etc.),
- – sanitation and environmental hygiene,
- – existing levels of immunity;
- Availability of effective preventive measures, including:
  - – immunization/preventive antisera,
  - – sanitation,
  - – vector and reservoir control;
- Availability of effective treatment, including:
  - – passive immunization,
  - – post-exposure vaccination,
  - – antimicrobials/chemotherapeutic agents (including any data on resistance patterns).

SAFE WORKING PRACTICES

The safety of the staff must be a prime consideration when a laboratory is set up. It is wholly unethical to expect staff to work in conditions where safety is ignored. The level of safety required has profound implications for the design and working of the laboratory.

Safe working in the laboratory depends on the observance of basic safety precautions (Table A9.1) and on good training of staff both in safety and in good bench work. The level of the safety precautions that may need to be established over and above the general safety principles will depend on:

- the types of tests to be done,
- the types of organism present and the risks they pose due to their pathogenicity, mode of transmission, etc.
- whether work higher risk work is appropriate at the local level.

The safety levels that can be achieved in a laboratory (and hence the types of test that can be offered) also depend on the possibility of maintaining and sustaining safety equipment.

Infectious microorganisms can be classified into four risk groups (Table A9.2) and the level of safety needed to handle them can then be determined (Table A9.3).

Table A9.1 **General safety principles**

- The laboratory should have a written manual of safe practice and this should be followed at all times.
- A first-aid box must be provided and a staff member trained in first aid should be present at all times when the laboratory is working.
- Eyewash facilities must be provided.
- Only the laboratory staff should be permitted to enter the working area of the laboratory.
- Laboratory staff should wear protective clothing, which should be removed when they leave the laboratory itself. It should not be worn in laboratory support areas such as offices, staff rooms, etc. Protective clothing should never be stored in the same lockers as street clothing.
- Appropriate shoes should be worn. Open-toed shoes (sandals) are not suitable for wear in the laboratory.
- Face protection (goggles/masks/eyeshields) should be provided and worn when procedures that may produce aerosols or splashes are undertaken.
- Rubber gloves should always be worn when handling specimens and they or other appropriate protective gloves should be worn for other hazardous procedures.
- Mouth pipetting should be absolutely forbidden.
- Hypodermic syringes and needles should not be used as pipetting devices.
- All contaminated material (specimens, glassware, sharps, etc) should be decontaminated before disposal or cleaning for re-use. To this end, appropriate containers (sharps bins, sealable plastic bags, disinfectant pots) and disinfectants must be provided.
- A predictable unidirectional airflow across and out of the laboratory should be maintained when the laboratory is in use (see "Ventilation" below).
- Eating, drinking, smoking and applying cosmetics should be forbidden in the laboratory.
- Laboratory staff should clean and disinfect all benches at the end of the working day or if infectious material is spilt.
- Laboratory staff should always wash their hands when leaving the laboratory and facilities must be provided for this purpose.
- All spills, accidents, etc. should be reported to the laboratory supervisor.

Table A9.2 **Infectious microorganisms classified by risk group**

Group	Risk	Definition
1	No or very low individual and community risk	A microorganism that is unlikely to cause animal or human disease
2	Moderate risk to individuals, low risk to the community	A pathogen that can cause human or animal disease but is unlikely to be a serious hazard to laboratory workers, the community, livestock or the environment. Laboratory exposures may cause serious infection but effective treatment and preventive measures are available and the risk of spread of infection is limited
3	High risk to individuals, low risk to the community	A pathogen that usually causes serious human or animal disease but does not ordinarily spread from one infected individual to another. Effective treatment and preventive measures are available.
4	High risk to individuals and the community	A pathogen that usually causes serious human or animal disease and that can be readily transmitted from one individual to another, directly or indirectly. Effective treatment and preventive measures are not usually available.

Table A9.3 **Risk groups, biosafety levels, laboratory practice and safety equipment**

Risk group	Biosafety level	Types of laboratories	Laboratory practice	Safety equipment
1	1 (basic)	Basic teaching	GMBT[a]	None. Open bench work
2	2 (basic)	Primary health services, primary level hospital diagnostic, teaching and public health services	GMBT + basic protective clothing; biohazard signs	Open bench + Class I or II BSC[b] for potential aerosols
3	3 (containment)	Special diagnostic	As level 2 + special protective clothing, controlled access, directional air flow	Class I or II BSC and/or other primary containment for all work
4	4 (maximum containment)	Dangerous pathogen units	As level 3 + airlock entry, shower exit, special waste disposal	Class III BSC or positive pressure suits, double ended autoclave, filtered air

[a] GMBT = good microbiological bench technique
[b] BSC = biological safety cabinet

Where toxic or corrosive chemicals are involved a suitable fume hood with an extractor fan will be required. Such equipment is not safe for work involving biological hazards. Where the work involves dangerous pathogens (risk group 2 and higher – Tables A8.2 and A8.3) properly designed safety cabinets will be required.

In general the type of laboratory that will be set up in the early stages of an emergency will be of basic level 1. However, in many areas where disasters occur there is a risk of exposure to organisms in the higher risk groups. This must be taken into account when the laboratory is set up. The tests that can be done may be limited by the potential risk. It is rare that high biosafety levels will be appropriate for a local laboratory in an emergency but it may well be that as a result some tests simply cannot be undertaken locally because safe working cannot be guaranteed.

EQUIPPING EMERGENCY LABORATORIES

The ability of a laboratory to perform even the most basic tests depends on the quality of its equipment. The equipment must not only be suitable for the tests required, it must also be safe. It should be designed with certain general principles in mind:

- It should prevent (or at least limit) contact between the operator and infectious material.
- It should be made from materials that are corrosion resistant, impermeable to liquids and sufficiently strong.
- It must be free of sharp edges and moving parts must be protected.
- It must be simple to install, operate, maintain, decontaminate and clean.
- It must be electrically safe.

Microscopes

Objective lens. This produces the initial (primary) image, which is then enlarged and focused by the eyepiece. The total magnification is the product of the magnification of these two lenses. The ability of the objective lens to differentiate fine detail is called its resolving power and is dependent on:

1. The "numerical aperture" (NA) of the lens (a factor of its diameter and focal length). The higher the NA the greater the resolving power. The NAs of the commonly used objectives for microscopes with the normal 160 mm tube lengths are: 10 x objective – NA 0.25

40 x objective – NA 0.65

100 x (oil) objective – NA 1.25

2. Correction for optical aberrations. The best objectives for general purposes are Achromats. Flat field (Plan) Achromats are additionally corrected so that the entire field is in focus but are more expensive.

Objectives should ideally be parfocal so that when the nosepiece of the microscope is revolved to bring a new objective into the light path no refocusing is needed. Modern objectives are produced to the DIN standard. These are longer than older objectives and should not be mixed with them, as they will not be parfocal. The use of such a mixture of lenses poses the risk of damaging or breaking the slide. The 40x and 100x objectives should also be spring-loaded to avoid damaging slides.

Oil immersion lenses. Significant loss of light and detail at high magnification can be avoided by filling the gap between the lens and the specimen with oil of the same optical properties as glass (immersion oil). The use of synthetic non-drying immersion oil is recommended.

The eyepiece allows the detail collected by the objective lens to be seen. Too great an eyepiece magnification can cause blurring of the image. Eyepieces of 10 x magnification are generally used but 7 x eyepieces are valuable for use with oil immersion lenses as the image, although smaller, is sharper. Microscopes can have one eyepiece (monocular) or two (binocular). The latter are more restful to use and the standard of microscopy is better.

Illumination. Microscopes generally have an integral controllable light source. Low-wattage halogen sources are best and give a consistent uniform light. (NB. The built-in illumination systems of cheaper microscopes may not be made to acceptable safety standards.) Where electricity supplies are likely to be intermittent (or non-existent), a microscope that can also take a mirror unit should be supplied.

Substage condenser. Allows the operator to manipulate the light impinging on the object. Ideally the light beam should be parallel to provide an even intensity over the whole image field. The intensity of the light beam can be altered with an iris diaphragm and focused by means of a focusing knob. Condensers should be of the Abbe type with a diaphragm and a swing-out filter holder. The condenser mount should allow the condenser to be centred by use of adjustment screws unless it has been pre-centred by the manufacturer.

Filters may be needed to reduce light intensity, to alter light colour (to affect the contrast of the image) or to transmit light of a particular wavelength (e.g. for fluorescence microscopy).

Mechanical stage. The microscope slide is supported on a platform called the stage. Ideally this should allow the slide to be moved (or the stage itself to be moved) by the use of two control wheels. A mechanical stage should have smooth-running controls and should be fitted with vernier scales so that specimens can easily be located. An integral mechanical stage is better than a "bolt on" version as it will be more robust.

Focusing controls must be smooth in action (especially the fine focus), robust and must not be subject to drift. Specialist microscopes may be needed for certain types of diagnostic test. For example, some parasitological work requires dark ground illumination with a special sub-stage condenser.

Transporting microscopes. If the microscope is to be transported around for field use at different sites, a special padded transport box will be needed. The boxes in which most microscopes are supplied just provide for storage in the laboratory, not for regular transport. As an alternative there are a number of compact microscopes that have been produced for field use and one of these may be suitable for the job – however, these are rather expensive and are less comfortable to use than the ordinary laboratory instrument.

Storage. Provide dust covers. In the tropics, if at all possible, store the microscope in a box with a low-wattage light bulb in it that is on all the time and with holes to allow air circulation. This will warm and dry the air in the box and prevent the growth of fungus on the lenses.

Local purchase. When considering where to buy microscopes, consider buying locally if this does not compromise quality. It could greatly ease supply of spares, maintenance, etc.

Centrifuges

Centrifuges may be required for:

- – measurement of haematocrit – packed cell volume (PCV),
- – separation of blood cells from plasma,
- – concentration of casts and cells in urine,
- – concentration of cells in CSF,
- – concentration of stool samples.

Two types of centrifuge are of value in the basic diagnostic laboratory. These are:

- *Haematocrit centrifuge.* These small but fast-spinning centrifuges are used for:
  - – measurement of haematocrit in the investigation of iron deficiency and other forms of anaemia,
  - – the microhaematocrit concentration technique for detecting motile trypanosomes and microfilariae.
- *General purpose bench centrifuge.* These are used for:
  - – sedimenting cells, parasites and bacteria in body fluids for microscopical examination,
  - – to wash red cells, obtain serum and perform cross matching,
  - – to concentrate parasites,
  - – to obtain plasma or serum for clinical chemistry and antibody tests.

Colorimeters and haemoglobinometers

Colorimeters are used for the quantitative determination of substances (such as haemoglobin and serum glucose) that can alter in concentration during disease and treatment. Haemoglobinometers can measure only haemoglobin.

Simple colorimeters such as Lovibond comparators (portable colorimeters that require no external power source) can be used for a number of basic biochemical tests. Battery-operated instruments are available for more accurate and sophisticated measurements.

Autoclaves and sterilization

Many activities in medical laboratories require the use of sterile equipment, media or fluids. Equally, laboratories may produce waste material that may need to be sterilized before it can be discarded. Autoclaving is a convenient way to sterilise items in the laboratory. Essentially it involves heating the items to up to 20 °C above the boiling point of water in a pressure vessel. This allows more rapid sterilization than simple boiling and also kills organisms (such as some bacterial spores) that are not killed by boiling. Autoclaves are quite sophisticated pieces of equipment and if only small amounts of small items need to be sterilized an ordinary domestic pressure cooker is quite adequate.

You will need autoclave indicator tape (with stripes that change colour above boiling water temperature) to mark items to ensure that the process is working satisfactorily.

Boiling water sterilizers are reasonably efficient but will not kill all pathogenic microorganisms (e.g. some bacterial spores are resistant to boiling but are killed by autoclaving).

Refrigerators

Refrigerators and freezers that run on gas or kerosene are available and the suitability of this type of equipment as compared with electric machines should be considered (dual fuel gas/electric refrigerators are of especial value in these situations).

Refrigerators are essential pieces of laboratory equipment in all but the most basic laboratories. There are two main types:

1. *Electrical compression* (The standard European refrigerator. They have a heat exchanger [on the back usually] of thin tubes – ca 0.5 cm – and a dumpy compressor at the bottom).

2. *Absorption* (have a heat exchanger [on the back usually] of thick tubes).

Compression refrigerators are electrical and require less energy to run than the absorption type. However absorption refrigerators are available that can run off gas, kerosene or electricity or dual fuels (e.g. electricity/gas). Selection should be based on available fuels. (NB. Solar refrigerators are available.)

Ice-lined refrigerators are useful where electricity supplies are intermittent, as they remain cold for hours even when there is no power. The holdover times of domestic refrigerators can be improved by putting some bottles filled with water near the top and by improving the insulation of the door. Open refrigerators as few times as possible especially if power is off so that loss of cold air is kept to a minimum.

Domestic refrigerators are not safe for the storage of flammable materials as they are not spark-protected.

Freezers may be needed for storage of critical reagents. Consider a refrigerator with a freezer compartment unless a large freezer capacity is required. You need to be aware that a refrigerator with a freezer compartment will use much more fuel than one without.

Refrigerators that open from the top are much more efficient than those with a front door. However the latter are much more common and tend therefore to be cheaper. It is also usually easier to find things in the latter.

Water purification systems

Many laboratory tests (e.g. preparing malaria slides) require pure water. There are a number of methods available for treating water for laboratory use:

Filtration removes suspended solids and other materials by passage through material with a small pore size. Ceramic filters will remove all potential pathogens except viruses. Filters do not remove dissolved chemicals.

Distillation removes non-volatile materials, solids and all inorganics. Stills require quite a lot of energy to heat them and a great deal of cool water to condense the distillate (at least 50 litres/hour at a supply pressure of 0.3 kg/cm^2). Many stills are made from glass and are fragile but stainless steel stills are available.

Demineralizers do not require energy input but they do not produce completely pure water. They use ion-absorbing resins remove inorganic ions and some organic materials from the water. They can become contaminated with bacteria and their ability to remove ions declines steadily unless they are well cared for and regenerated. Portable demineralizers are available for small-scale use.

Reverse osmosis produces good-quality water but is energy-intensive and the membranes used are easily damaged.

Removal of suspended solids can be achieved by settlement (allow the water to stand overnight and remove the supernatant) or by adding aluminium sulfate to the water at the rate of 5 g to 10 litres of water, allowing to stand for 20 minutes and pouring off the clear supernatant. This dose not produce pure water but does remove many contaminants and is an essential prerequisite for the use of equipment such as reverse osmosis machines and filters.

Adjustment of pH. Water for laboratory use should have a neutral pH of 7.0. Measure pH with a meter or with pH paper strips. Dilute hydrochloric acid can be used to lower pH and dilute sodium hydroxide to raise it.

Filtration and/or demineralization is a good way to provide reasonable amounts of adequately pure water for laboratory use especially in areas where water supplies and/or electricity supplies are unreliable.

Measurement of pH

Many basic laboratory processes require buffered solutions or solutions of known pH; pH can be measured simply by means of special indicator papers but a more satisfactory method is to use a pH meter. These can be battery or mains operated. Chose a pH meter that will measure the whole pH range (0–14) and that has automatic temperature compensation.

Incinerators

Plans for a basic incinerator suitable for emergency use can be found in *health laboratory facilities in emergency and disaster situations*. Plans for a more sophisticated plant are given in *Engineering in emergencies*.

REFERENCES

Basic Laboratory Methods in Medical Parasitology. Geneva, World Health Organization, 1991.

Bench Aids for the diagnosis of malaria infections. (2nd Edition). Geneva, World Health Organization, 2000.

Bench Aids for the diagnosis of filarial infections. Geneva, World Health Organization, 1997.

Bench Aids for the diagnosis of intestinal parasites. Geneva, World Health Organization, 1994.

Guidelines for the Collection of Clinical Specimens during Field Investigation of Outbreaks. Geneva, World Health Organization, 2000 (document WHO/CDS/CSR/EDC/2000.4).

Health laboratory facilities in emergency and disaster situations. Alexandria, World Health Organization Regional Office for the Eastern Mediterranean, 1994 (document WHO/EMRO No. 6).

Laboratory Biosafety Manual. (2nd Edition). Geneva, World Health Organization, 1993.

Maintenance and repair of laboratory Diagnostic, Imaging and Hospital Equipment. Geneva, World Health Organization, 1994.

Safety in Health-Care Laboratories. Geneva, World Health Organization, 1997.

Selection of Basic Laboratory Equipment for Laboratories with Limited Resources. Alexandria, World Health Organization Regional Office for the Eastern Mediterranean, 2000.

Other relevant publications

Cheesbrough M. *Laboratory practice in tropical countries. Part 1.* Cambridge, Cambridge University Press, 1998.

Cheesbrough M. *Laboratory practice in tropical countries. Part 2* Cambridge, Cambridge University Press, 2000.

Médecins Sans Frontières. *Refugee health.* London, Macmillan, 1997.

10. Treatment guidelines

These treatment guidelines are intended to give simple guidance for the training of primary health care workers, using basic units of New Emergency Health Kits. In the dosage guidelines, five age groups have been distinguished, except for the treatment of diarrhoea with oral rehydration fluid where six age and weight categories are used. When dosage is shown as "1 tab × 2", one tablet should be taken in the morning and one before bedtime. When dosage is shown as "2 tab × 3", two tablets should be taken in the morning, two in the middle of the day and two before bedtime. These guidelines have been adapted from *The new emergency health kit 98* which is currently under review.[8]

The treatment guidelines contain the following diagnostic/symptom groups:
- anaemia,
- pain,
- diarrhoea,
- fever,
- preventive care in pregnancy,
- measles,
- respiratory tract infections,
- worms,
- skin conditions,
- eyes,
- sexually transmitted and urinary tract infections.

Anaemia

Diagnosis Symptom	Weight	$0 \leq 4$ kg	$4 \leq 8$ kg	$8 \leq 15$ kg	$15 \leq 35$ kg	35 kg +
	Age	$0 \leq 2$ months	2 months $\leq$ 1 year	$1 \leq 5$ years	$5 \leq 15$ years	15 years +
Severe anaemia (oedema, dizziness, shortness of breath)		**Refer**				
Moderate anaemia (pallor and tiredness)		**Refer**	Ferrous sulfate + folic acid, 1 tab daily for at least 2 months	Ferrous sulfate + folic acid, 2 tab daily for at least 2 months	Ferrous sulfate + folic acid, 3 tab daily for at least 2 months	Ferrous sulfate + folic acid, 3 tab daily for at least 2 months

---

8 *The new emergency health kit 98.* Geneva, World Health Organization, 1998 (document WHO/DAP/98.10), under review.

Pain

Diagnosis Symptom	Weight	0 ≤ 4 kg	4 ≤ 8 kg	8 ≤ 15 kg	15 ≤ 35 kg	35 kg +
	Age	0 ≤ 2 months	2 months ≤ 1 year	1 ≤ 5 years	5 ≤ 15 years	15 years +
Pain (headache, joint pain, toothache)			Paracetamol, tablet 100 mg, 1/2 tab × 3	Paracetamol, tablet 100 mg, 1 tab × 3	ASA,[a,b] tab 300 mg, 1 tab × 3	ASA, tablet 300 mg, 2 tab × 3
Stomach pain				**Refer**	Aluminium hydroxide, 1/2 tab × 3 for 3 days	Aluminium hydroxide, 1 tab × 3 for 3 days

[a] *ASA = acetylsalicylic acid.*
[b] *For children under 12 years, paracetamol is preferred because of the risk of Reye syndrome.*

Diarrhoea

Diagnosis Symptom	Weight	0 ≤ 5 kg	5–7.9 kg	8–10.9 kg	11–15.9 kg	16–29.9 kg	30 kg +
	Age[a]	< 4 months	4–11 months	12–23 months	2–4 years	5–14 years	15 years +
Diarrhoea with some dehydration (WHO Treatment Plan B)[b]		Approximate amount of ORS solution to give in the first 4 hours (in ml)					
		200–400	400–600	600–800	800–1200	1200–2200	2200–4000
Diarrhoea lasting more than two weeks or in malnourished patient or patient in poor condition		Give ORS according to dehydration stage and **refer**					
Bloody diarrhoea[c] (check presence of blood in stools)		Give ORS according to dehydration stage and **refer**					
Diarrhoea with severe dehydration (WHO Treatment Plan C)[d]		**Refer** patient for nasogastric tube and/or intravenous treatment					
Diarrhoea with no dehydration (WHO Treatment Plan A)[e]		Continue to feed Advise the patient to return to the health worker in case of frequent stools, increased thirst, sunken eyes or fever; or when the patient does not eat or drink normally; or does not get better within three days; or develops blood in the stool or repeated vomiting					

[a] Use the patient's age only when you do not know the weight. The approximate amount of ORS required (in ml) can also be calculated by multiplying the patient's weight (in grams) times 0.075.
[b] *The new emergency health kit 98*, Annex 2c.
[c] Protocol to be established according to epidemiological data.
[d] *The new emergency health kit 98*, Annex 2d.
[e] *The new emergency health kit 98*, Annex 2b.

Use of drugs for children with diarrhoea

- **Antimicrobial** should be used only for dysentery and for suspected cases of cholera with severe dehydration. Otherwise they are ineffective and should **not** be given.

- **Antiparasitic drugs** should be used **only** for:
  - amoebiasis, after antimicrobial treatment of bloody diarrhoea for *Shigella* has failed, or trophozoites of *Entamoeba histolytica* containing red blood cells are seen in the faeces;
  - giardiasis, when diarrhoea has lasted for at least 14 days **and** cysts or trophozoites of *Giardia* are seen in the faeces or small bowel fluid.

- **Antidiarrhoeal drugs** and **anti-emetics** should **never** be used. None has any proven value and some are dangerous.

Fever

Diagnosis Symptom	Weight	0 ≤ 4 kg	4 ≤ 8 kg	8 ≤ 15 kg	15 ≤ 35 kg	35 kg +
	Age	0 ≤ 2 months	2 months ≤ 1 year	1 ≤ 5 years	5 ≤ 15 years	15 years +
Fever in malnourished patient or patient in poor condition, or when in doubt		Refer				
Fever with chills, presumed malaria		Refer	Check national protocols and WHO recommendations			
Fever with cough		**Refer**	See "Respiratory tract infections" below			
Fever (unspecified)		**Refer**	Paracetamol, tab 100 mg, 1/2 tab × 3 for 1 to 3 days	Paracetamol, tab 100 mg, 1 tab × 3 for 1–3 days	ASA,[b,c] tab 300 mg, 1 tab × 3 for 1–3 days	ASA, tab 300 mg, 2 tab × 3 for 1–3 days

[a] *First-, second- and third-line therapies will vary according to resistance patterns in the country – check national protocols and WHO recommendations (see Section 5.12 on malaria).*

[b] *ASA = acetylsalicylic acid.*

[c] *For children under 12 years, paracetamol is to be preferred because of the risk of Reye syndrome.*

Preventive care in pregnancy

Diagnosis Symptom	Weight	$0 \leq 4$ kg	$4 \leq 8$ kg	$8 \leq 15$ kg	$15 \leq 35$ kg	35 kg +
	Age	$0 \leq 2$ months	2 months $\leq$ 1 year	$1 \leq 5$ years	$5 \leq 15$ years	15 years +
Anaemia (for treatment see under Anaemia)						Ferrous sulfate + folic acid, 1 tab daily throughout pregnancy
Malaria (for treatment see under Fever)						SP: 3 tab twice at least, during pregnancy: once during 2nd trimester and one during 3rd trimester[a]

[a] *See malaria Section 5.12 for recommendations on pregnancy and HIV.* **Consult national protocols and WHO recommendations.**

Measles

Diagnosis Symptom	Weight	$0 \leq 4$ kg	$4 < 8$ kg	$8 \leq 15$ kg	$15 \leq 35$ kg	35 kg +
	Age	$0 \leq 2$ months	2 months $\leq$ 1 year	$1 \leq 5$ years	$5 \leq 15$ years	15 years +
Measles			Treat respiratory tract disease according to symptoms Treat conjunctivitis as "red eyes" Treat diarrhoea according to symptoms Continue (breast)feeding, give retinol (vitamin A)			

Respiratory tract infections

Diagnosis Symptom	Weight / Age	0 ≤ 4 kg / 0 ≤ 2 months	4 ≤ 8 kg / 2 months ≤ 1 year	8 ≤ 15 kg / 1 ≤ 5 years	15 ≤ 35 kg / 5 ≤ 15 years	35 kg + / 15 years +
Severe pneumonia[a]		Give the first dose of co-trimoxazole (see under Pneumonia) and **refer**				
Pneumonia[a]	**Refer**	Co-trimoxazole, tab 400 mg SMX[a] + 80 mg TMP,[b] 1/2 tab × 2 for 5 days	Co-trimoxazole, tab 400 mg SMX + 80 mg TMP, 1 tab × 2 for 5 days	Co-trimoxazole, tab 400 mg SMX + 80 mg TMP, 1 tab × 2 for 5 days	Co-trimoxazole, tab 400 mg SMX + 80 mg TMP, 2 tab × 2 for 5 days
		Reassess after 2 days; continue (breast)feeding, give fluids, clear the nose; return if breathing becomes faster or more difficult, or not able to drink or if the condition deteriorates.				
No pneumonia: cough or cold[a]	**Refer**	Paracetamol[c] tab 100 mg 1/2 tab × 3 for 1–3 days	Paracetamol tab 100 mg 1 tab × 3 for 1–3 days	ASA[d,e] tab 300 mg 1 tab × 3 for 1–3 days	ASA tab 300 mg 2 tab × 3 for 1–3 days
		Supportive therapy; continue (breast)feeding, give fluids, clear the nose; return if breathing becomes faster or more difficult, or not able to drink or if the condition deteriorates.				
Prolonged cough (30 days)	**Refer**					
Acute ear pain and/or ear discharge for less than 2 weeks	**Refer**	Co-trimoxazole, tab 400 mg SMX + 80 mg TMP, 1/2 tab × 2 for 5 days	Co-trimoxazole, tab 400 mg SMX + 80 mg TMP 1 tab × 2 for 5 days	Co-trimoxazole, tab 400 mg SMX + 80 mg TMP 1 tab × 2 for 5 days	Co-trimoxazole, tab 400 mg SMX + 80 mg TMP 2 tab × 2 for 5 days
Ear discharge for more than 2 weeks, no pain or fever		Clean the ear once daily by syringe without needle using lukewarm clean water. Repeat until the water comes out clean. Dry repeatedly with clean piece of cloth.				

[a] *SMX = sulfamethoxazole.*
[b] *TMP = trimethoprim.*
[c] *If fever is present.*
[d] *ASA = acetylsalicylic acid.*
[e] *For children under 12 years, paracetamol is to be preferred because of the risk of Reye syndrome.*

Worms[a]

	Weight	0 ≤ 4 kg	4 ≤ 8 kg	8 ≤ 15 kg	15 ≤ 35 kg	35 kg +
Diagnosis Symptom	Age	0 ≤ 2 months	2 months ≤ 1 year	1 ≤ 5 years	5 ≤ 15 years	15 years +
Roundworm, pinworm				Mebendazole, tab 100 mg, 2 tab once	Mebendazole, tab 100 mg, 2 tab once	Mebendazole, tab 100 mg, 2 tab once
Hookworm				Mebendazole, tab 100 mg, 1 tab × 2 for 3 days	Mebendazole, tab 100 mg, 1 tab × 2 for 3 days	Mebendazole, tab 100 mg, 1 tab × 2 for 3 days

[a] *Treatment of hookworm in pregnancy with mebendazole is recommended in endemic areas; mebendazole can safely be given in the second and third trimesters of pregnancy.*

Skin conditions

Wounds: extensive, deep or on face	**Refer**
Wounds: limited and superficial	Clean with clean water and soap or **diluted** chlorhexidine solution;[a] gently apply gentian violet solution [b] once a day
Severe burns (on face or extensive)	Treat as for mild burns and **refer**
Mild to moderate burns	Immerse **immediately** in cold water, or use a cold wet cloth; continue until pain eases, then treat as for wounds
Severe bacterial infection (with fever)	**Refer**
Mild bacterial infection	Clean with clean water and soap or **diluted** chlorhexidine solution Apply gentian violet solution twice a day If not improved after 10 days, **refer**
Fungal infection	Apply gentian violet solution once a day for 5 days
Infected scabies	Bacterial infection: clean with clean water and soap or **diluted** chlorhexidine solution Apply gentian violet solution twice a day when infection is cured:
	children < 12 years: apply **diluted** benzyl benzoate[c] once a day for 3 days children ≥ 12 years and adults: apply **non-diluted** benzyl benzoate (25%) once a day for 3 days
Non-infected scabies	children < 12 years: apply **diluted** benzyl benzoate[c] once a day for 3 days children ≥ 12 years and adults: apply **non-diluted** benzyl benzoate (25%) once a day for 3 days

[a] *Chlorhexidine 5% must always be diluted before use: 20 ml made up to 1 litre with water. Take the 1-litre plastic bottle supplied with the kit; put 20 ml of chlorhexidine solution into the bottle using the 10-ml syringe supplied and fill up the bottle with boiled or clean water. Chlorhexidine 1.5% + cetrimide 15% solution should be used in the same dilution.*

[b] *Gentian violet 0.5% concentration = 1 teaspoon of gentian violet powder per litre of boiled/clean water. Shake well, or use warm water to dissolve all the powder.*

[c] *Children 1–12 years, at half strength (12.5%): dilute by mixing 0.5 litre benzyl benzoate 25% with 0.5 litre clean water in the 1-litre bottle supplied with the kit. Infants (0–12 months), at quarter strength (6.25%): dilute by mixing 0.5 litre benzyl benzoate 12.5% with 0.5 litre clean water.*

Eyes

Red eyes (conjunctivitis)	Apply tetracycline eye ointment 3 times a day for 7 days. If not improved after 3 days or in doubt, **refer**.

Sexually transmitted and urinary tract infections

Suspicion of sexually transmitted or urinary tract infection	**Refer**

11. Management of the child with cough or difficulty in breathing[9]

1. ASSESS THE CHILD

Ask

- How old is the child?
- Is the child coughing? For how long?
- Is the child able to drink (for children age 2 months up to 5 years)?
- Has the young infant stopped feeding well (for children less than 2 months)?
- Has the child had fever? For how long?
- Has the child had convulsions?

Look and listen (the child must be calm)

- Count the breaths in a minute.
- Look for chest indrawing.
- Look and listen for stridor.
- Look and listen for wheeze. Is it recurrent?
- See whether the child is abnormally sleepy, or difficult to wake.
- Feel for fever, or low body temperature (or measure temperature).
- Look for severe undernutrition.

2 DECIDE HOW TO TREAT THE CHILD

The child aged less than 2 months: *see Table A11.1*

The child aged 2 months up to 5 years:

- who is not wheezing: *see Table A11.2*
- who is wheezing: *refer*

Treatment instructions: *see Table A11.3*

- give an antimicrobial
- advise mother to give home care
- treat fever

---

[9] *Source: Integrated management of childhood illness.* Geneva, World Health Organization, 1997.

Table A11.1 Child under 2 months of age

Signs	No fast breathing (less than 60 per minute) and No severe chest indrawing	Fast breathing (60 per minute or more) or Severe chest indrawing	Not able to drink Convulsions Abnormally sleepy or difficult to wake Stridor in calm child Wheezing or Fever or low body temperature
Classification	No pneumonia – cough or cold	Severe pneumonia	Very severe disease
Treatment	Advise mother to give following home care: - keep infant warm - breastfeed frequently - clear nose if it interferes with feeding Advise mother to return quickly if: - illness worsens - breathing is difficult - breathing becomes fast - feeding becomes a problem	Refer urgently to hospital Give first dose of an antimicrobial Keep infant warm (If referral is not feasible, treat with an antimicrobial and follow closely)	Refer urgently to hospital Give first dose of an antimicrobial Keep infant warm (If referral is not feasible, treat with an antimicrobial and follow closely)

Table A11.2 **Child 2 months to 5 years of age**

Signs	No chest indrawing and No fast breathing (less than 50 per minute if child 2–12 months of age or 40 per minute if child 1–5 years)	No chest indrawing and Fast breathing (50 per minute or more if child 2–12 months of age or 40 per minute if child 1–5 years)	Chest indrawing	Not able to drink Convulsions Abnormally sleepy or difficult to wake Stridor in calm child or Severe undernutrition
Classification	No pneumonia – cough or cold	Pneumonia	Severe pneumonia	Very severe disease
Treatment	If coughing more than 30 days, **refer** for assessment Assess and treat ear problem or sore throat if present Assess and treat other problems Advise mother to give home care Treat fever if present	Advise mother to give home care Give an antimicrobial Treat fever if present Advise mother to return in 2 days for reassessment, or if the child is getting worse	**Refer** urgently to hospital Give first dose of antimicrobial Treat fever if present (If referral is not possible, treat with an antimicrobial and follow closely)	**Refer** urgently to hospital Give first dose of antimicrobial Treat fever if present If cerebral malaria is possible, give an antimalarial drug

Reassess in 2 days a child who is taking an antimicrobial for pneumonia			
Signs	**Improving** • Less fever • Eating better • Breathing slower	**The same**	**Worse** • Not able to drink • Has chest indrawing • Has other danger signs
Treatment	Finish 5 days of antimicrobial	Change antimicrobial or **Refer**	**Refer** urgently to hospital

Table A11.3 Treatment instructions

- Give an antimicrobial.

- Give first dose of antimicrobial in the clinic.

- Instruct mother on how to give the antimicrobial for 5 days at home (or to return to clinic for daily procaine penicillin injection):

Age or weight	Co-trimoxazole: trimethoprim (TMP) + sulfamethoxazole (SMX)			Amoxicillin		Procaine penicillin
	Twice daily for 5 days			Three times daily for 5 days		Once daily for 5 days
	Adult tablet single strength (80 mg TMP + 400 mg SMX)	Paediatric tablet (20 mg TMP + 100 mg SMX)	Syrup (40 mg TMP + 200 mg SMX)	Tablet (250 mg)	Syrup (125 mg in 5 ml)	Intramuscular injection
Under 2 months (< 6 kg)[a]	1/4 [b]	1 [b]	2.5 ml[b]	1/4	2.5 ml	200 000 units
2 months – 12 months (6–9 kg)	1/2	2	5.0 ml	1/2	5.0 ml	400 000 units
12 months – 5 years (10–19 kg)	1	3	7.5 ml	1	10 ml	800 000 units

[a] *Give oral antimicrobial for five days at home if referral is not feasible.*

[b] *If the child is less than one month old, give 1/2 paediatric tablet or 1.25 ml syrup twice daily. Avoid co-trimoxazole in infants under one month of age who are premature or jaundiced. Syrups and paediatric tablets are mentioned here for the sake of completeness; they are not available in the kit.*

Advise mother to give home care (for child aged 2 months to 5 years):
- Feed the child:
  - feed the child during illness
  - increase feeding during illness
  - clear the nose if it interferes with feeding
- Increase fluids:
  - offer the child extra to drink
  - increase breastfeeding
  - soothe the throat and relieve cough with a safe remedy

- **Most important**: for the child classified as having no pneumonia, cough or cold, watch for the following signs and return quickly if they occur:
  - breathing becomes difficult
  - breathing becomes fast   ➡ **This child may have pneumonia**
  - child not able to drink
  - child becomes sicker

- Treat fever:

Fever is high (> 39 °C)	Fever is not high (38–39 °C)
↓	
Give paracetamol	Advise mother to give more fluids

In falciparum malarious area: any fever **or** history of fever
↓
Give an antimalarial (or treat according to your national malaria programme recommendations)

Fever for more than 5 days
↓
Refer for assessment

Paracetamol dose every 6 hours		
Age or weight	100-mg tablet	500-mg tablet
2 months to 12 months (6–9 kg)	1	1/4
12 months to 3 years (10–14 kg)	1	1/4
3 years to 5 years (15–19 kg)	11/2	1/2

Fever for more than 5 days
Refer for assessment

12. Assessment and treatment of diarrhoea

Table A12.1 **Assessment of diarrhoeal patients for dehydration**

	PLAN A	PLAN B	PLAN C
First assess your patient for dehydration			
1. Look at: General condition	Well, alert	*Restless, irritable	*Lethargic or unconscious; floppy
Eyes[a]	Normal	Sunken	Very sunken and dry
Tears	Present	Absent	Absent
Mouth and tongue[b]	Moist	Dry	Very dry
Thirst	Drinks normally, not thirsty	*Thirsty, drinks eagerly	*Drinks poorly or not able to drink
2. Feel: Skin pinch[c]	Goes back quickly	*Goes back slowly	*Goes back very slowly
3. Decide	The patient has *no signs of dehydration*	If the patient has two or more signs, including at least one *sign there is *some dehydration*	If the patient has two or more signs, including at least one *sign there is *severe dehydration*
4. Treat	Use Treatment Plan A	Weigh the patient if possible and use Treatment Plan B	Weigh the patient and use Treatment Plan C **URGENTLY**

[a] *In some infants and children the eyes normally appear somewhat sunken. It is helpful to ask the mother if the child's eyes are normal or more sunken than usual.*

[b] *Dryness of the mouth and tongue can also be palpated with a clean finger. The mouth may always be dry in a child who habitually breathes through the mouth. The mouth may be wet in a dehydrated patient owing to recent vomiting or drinking.*

[c] *The skin pinch is less useful in infants or children with marasmus (severe wasting) or kwashiorkor (severe undernutrition with oedema) or in obese children.*

Source: *The treatment of diarrhoea: a manual for physicians and other senior health workers.* Geneva, World Health Organization, 1995 (document WHO/CDR/95.3).

TREATMENT PLAN A: TO TREAT DIARRHOEA AT HOME

Use this plan to teach the mother to:

- continue to treat at home her child's current episode of diarrhoea,
- give early treatment for future episodes of diarrhoea.

Explain the three rules for treating diarrhoea at home.

1. Give the child more fluids than usual to prevent dehydration

- Use recommended home fluids. These include: ORS solution, food-based fluids (such as soup, rice water and yoghurt drinks) and plain water. Use ORS solution as described in the box below.

  (Note: if the child is under 6 months of age and not yet taking solid food, give ORS solution or water rather than food-based fluid.)

- Give as much of these fluids as the child will take. Use the amounts shown below for ORS as a guide.
- Continue giving these fluids until the diarrhoea stops.

2. Give the child plenty of food to prevent undernutrition

- Continue to breastfeed frequently.
- If the child is not breastfed, give the usual milk.
- If the child is 6 months or older, or already taking solid food:
  - also give cereal or another starchy food mixed, if possible, with pulses, vegetables and meat or fish; add one or two teaspoonfuls of vegetable oil to each serving;
  - give fresh fruit juice or mashed banana to provide potassium;
  - give freshly prepared foods; cook and mash or grind food well;
  - encourage the child to eat: offer food at least six times a day;
  - give the same food after diarrhoea stops, and give an extra meal each day for 2 weeks.

3. Take the child to the health worker if he/she does not get better in 3 days or develops any of the following:

- many watery stools
- repeated vomiting
- marked thirst
- eating or drinking poorly
- fever
- blood in the stool

Children should be given ORS solutions at home if:

- they have been on Treatment Plan B or C;
- they cannot return to the health worker if the diarrhoea gets worse; or
- if it is national policy to give ORS to all children who see a health worker for diarrhoea.

If the child is to be given ORS solution at home, show the mother how much ORS to give after each loose stool and give her enough packets for 2 days.

Age	Amount of ORS to be given after each loose stool	Amount of ORS to provide for use at home
Under 24 months	50–100 ml	500 ml/day
2–10 years	100–200 ml	1000 ml/day
10 years or more	as much as wanted	2000 ml/day

- Describe and show the amount to be given after each stool, using a local measure.

Show the mother how to mix and to give ORS

- Give a teaspoonful every 1–2 minutes for a child under 2 years.
- Give frequent sips from a cup for older children.
- If the child vomits, wait 10 minutes. Then give the solution more slowly (for example, a spoonful every 2–3 minutes).
- If diarrhoea continues after the ORS packets are used up, tell the mother to give other fluids as described in the first rule above or return for more ORS.

TREATMENT PLAN B: TO TREAT DEHYDRATION

Table A12.2 **Approximate amount of ORS solution to give in the first 4 hours**

	Age[a]					
	< 4 months	4–11 months	12–23 months	2–4 years	5–14 years	15 years +
Weight	0 ≤ 5 kg	5–7.9 kg	8–10.9 kg	11–15.9 kg	16–29.9 kg	30 kg +
in ml	200–400	400–600	600–800	800–1200	1200–2200	2200–4000
in local measure						

[a] *Patient's age, only when you do not know the weight. The approximate amount of ORS required (in ml) can also be calculated by multiplying the patient's weight (in grams) times 0.075.*

- If the child wants more ORS than shown, give more.
- Encourage the mother to continue breastfeeding.
- For infants under 6 months who are not breastfed, also give 100–200 ml clean water during this period.

Observe the child carefully and help the mother give ORS solution.

- Show her how much solution to give the child.
- Show her how to give it – a teaspoonful every 1–2 minutes for a child under 2 years, frequent sips from a cup for an older child.
- Check from time to time to see if there are problems.
- If the child vomits, wait 10 minutes and then continue giving ORS, but more slowly, for example, a spoonful every 2–3 minutes.
- If the child's eyelids become puffy, stop the ORS and give plain water or breast milk. Give ORS according to Plan A when the puffiness is gone.

After 4 hours, reassess the child using the assessment chart, then select Plan A, B or C to continue treatment

- If there are no signs of dehydration, shift to Plan A. When dehydration has been corrected, the child usually passes urine and may also be tired and fall asleep.
- If signs indicating some dehydration are still present, repeat Plan B but start to offer food, milk and juice as described in Plan A.
- If signs indicating severe dehydration have appeared, shift to Plan C.

If the mother must leave before completing Treatment Plan B:

- Show her how much ORS to give to finish the 4-hour treatment at home.
- Give her enough ORS packets to complete rehydration, and for 2 more days as shown in Plan A.
- Show her how to prepare ORS solution.
- Explain to her the three rules in Plan A for treating her child at home:
    - to give ORS or other fluids until diarrhoea stops,
    - to feed the child,
    - to bring the child back to the health worker, if necessary.

TREATMENT PLAN C: TO TREAT SEVERE DEHYDRATION QUICKLY

Follow the arrows. If the answer is "yes" go across. If "no" go down.

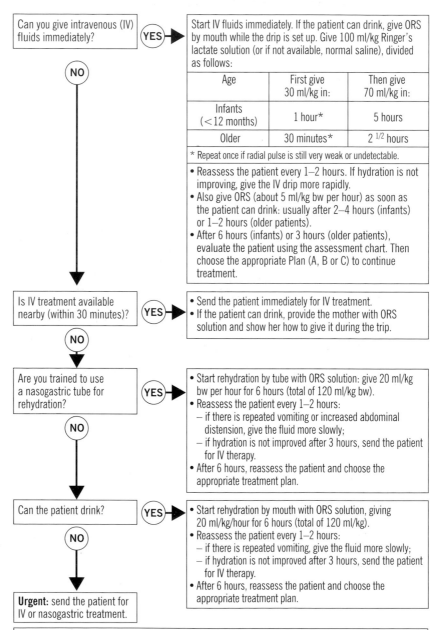

Can you give intravenous (IV) fluids immediately?

YES → Start IV fluids immediately. If the patient can drink, give ORS by mouth while the drip is set up. Give 100 ml/kg Ringer's lactate solution (or if not available, normal saline), divided as follows:

Age	First give 30 ml/kg in:	Then give 70 ml/kg in:
Infants (<12 months)	1 hour*	5 hours
Older	30 minutes*	2 1/2 hours

* Repeat once if radial pulse is still very weak or undetectable.

- Reassess the patient every 1–2 hours. If hydration is not improving, give the IV drip more rapidly.
- Also give ORS (about 5 ml/kg bw per hour) as soon as the patient can drink: usually after 2–4 hours (infants) or 1–2 hours (older patients).
- After 6 hours (infants) or 3 hours (older patients), evaluate the patient using the assessment chart. Then choose the appropriate Plan (A, B or C) to continue treatment.

NO ↓

Is IV treatment available nearby (within 30 minutes)? **YES** →
- Send the patient immediately for IV treatment.
- If the patient can drink, provide the mother with ORS solution and show her how to give it during the trip.

NO ↓

Are you trained to use a nasogastric tube for rehydration? **YES** →
- Start rehydration by tube with ORS solution: give 20 ml/kg bw per hour for 6 hours (total of 120 ml/kg bw).
- Reassess the patient every 1–2 hours:
  - if there is repeated vomiting or increased abdominal distension, give the fluid more slowly;
  - if hydration is not improved after 3 hours, send the patient for IV therapy.
- After 6 hours, reassess the patient and choose the appropriate treatment plan.

NO ↓

Can the patient drink? **YES** →
- Start rehydration by mouth with ORS solution, giving 20 ml/kg/hour for 6 hours (total of 120 ml/kg).
- Reassess the patient every 1–2 hours:
  - if there is repeated vomiting, give the fluid more slowly;
  - if hydration is not improved after 3 hours, send the patient for IV therapy.
- After 6 hours, reassess the patient and choose the appropriate treatment plan.

NO ↓

Urgent: send the patient for IV or nasogastric treatment.

If possible, observe the patient for at least 6 hours after rehydration to be sure the mother can maintain hydration giving ORS solution by mouth. If the patient is older than 2 years and there is cholera in the area, give an appropriate oral antimicrobial after the patient has become alert.

13. Flowcharts for syndromic management of sexually transmitted infections

A. URETHRAL DISCHARGE

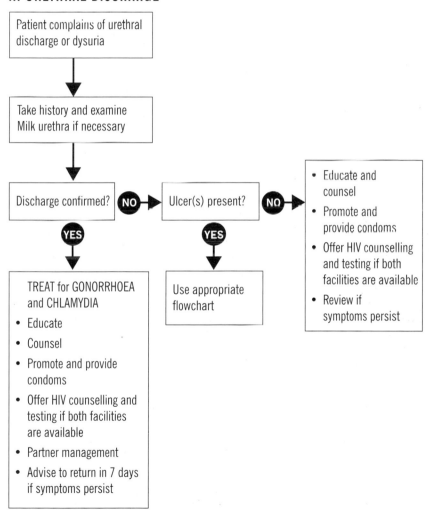

Source: *Guidelines for the management of sexually transmitted infections.* Geneva, World Health Organization, 2001 (document WHO/RHR/01.10).

B. GENITAL ULCERS

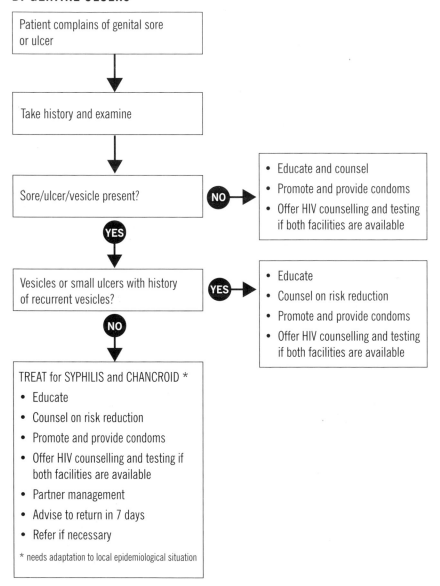

Patient complains of genital sore or ulcer

↓

Take history and examine

↓

Sore/ulcer/vesicle present? — **NO** →
- Educate and counsel
- Promote and provide condoms
- Offer HIV counselling and testing if both facilities are available

YES ↓

Vesicles or small ulcers with history of recurrent vesicles? — **YES** →
- Educate
- Counsel on risk reduction
- Promote and provide condoms
- Offer HIV counselling and testing if both facilities are available

NO ↓

TREAT for SYPHILIS and CHANCROID *
- Educate
- Counsel on risk reduction
- Promote and provide condoms
- Offer HIV counselling and testing if both facilities are available
- Partner management
- Advise to return in 7 days
- Refer if necessary

* needs adaptation to local epidemiological situation

Source: Guidelines for the management of sexually transmitted infections. Geneva, World Health Organization, 2001 (document WHO/RHR/01.10).

C. VAGINAL DISCHARGE

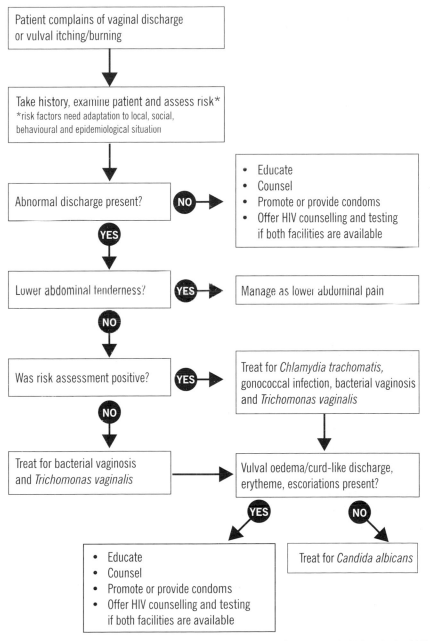

Source: Guidelines for the management of sexually transmitted infections. Geneva, World Health Organization, 2001 (document WHO/RHR/01.10).

14. Health card

HEALTH CARD
CARTE DE SANTÉ

Card No.
Carte N°

Date of registration
Date d'enregistrement

Date of arrival at site
Date d'arrivée sur le lieu

Site
Lieu

Section/House No.
Section / Habitation N°

Family name
Nom de famille

Given names
Prénoms

Date of birth or age
Date de naissance ou âge

or Years
ou Ans

Sex
Sexe

M / F

Name commonly known by
Nom d'usage habituel

Mother's name
Nom de la mère

Father's name
Nom du père

Height
Taille

cm

Weight
Poids

kg

Percentage weight/height
Pourcentage poids/taille

CHILDREN
ENFANTS

Feeding programme
Programme d'alimentation

Vaccination

Measles   Date
Rougeole

1

2

BCG
Date

Others
Autres

Polio   Date

DPT Polio   Date
DTC Polio

1

2

3

WOMEN
FEMMES

Pregnant   Yes/No
Enceinte   Oui/Non

No. of pregnancies
N° de grossesses

No. of children
N° d'enfants

Lactating   Yes/No
Allaitante   Oui/Non

Tetanus   Date
Tétanos

1

2

3

4

5

Feeding programme
Programme d'alimentation

COMMENTS
OBSERVATIONS

General (Family circumstances, living conditions, etc.)
Générales (Circonstances familiales, conditions de vie, etc.)

Health (Brief history, present condition)
Médicales (Résumé de l'état actuel)

DATE	CONDITION (Signs/symptoms/diagnosis) ETAT (Signes/symptômes/diagnostic)	TREATMENT (Medication/dose time) TRAITEMENT (Médication/durée de la dose)	COURSES (Medication due/given) APPLICATION (Médication requise/effectuée)	OBSERVATIONS (Change in condition) Name of health worker OBSERVATIONS (Changement d'état) Nom de l'agent de santé

Source: The New Emergency Health Kit 98. Geneva, World Health Organization, 1998 (document WHO/DAP/93.10).

15. List of WHO guidelines on communicable diseases

FACT SHEETS

Title	Publication No./Date
Anthrax	Fact Sheet No. 264 October 2001 http://www.who.int/mediacentre/factsheets/fs264/en/
Cholera	Fact Sheet No. 107 Revised March 2000 http://www.who.int/mediacentre/factsheets/fs107/en
Dengue and dengue haemorrhagic fever	Fact Sheet No. 117 Revised April 2002 http://www.who.int/mediacentre/factsheets/fs117/en/
Diphtheria	Fact Sheet No. 89 Revised December 2000 http://www.who.int/mediacentre/factsheets/fs089/en/
Food safety and foodborne illness	Fact Sheet No. 237 revised January 2002 http://www.who.int/mediacentre/factsheets/fs237/en/
Hepatitis B	Fact Sheet No. 204 Revised October 2000 http://www.who.int/mediacentre/factsheets/fs204/en/
Hepatitis C	Fact Sheet No. 164 Revised October 2000 http://www.who.int/mediacentre/factsheets/fs164/en/
Influenza	Fact Sheet No. 211 March 2003 http://www.who.int/mediacentre/factsheets/fs211/en/
Injection safety: background	Fact Sheet No. 231 Revised April 2002 http://www.who.int/mediacentre/factsheets/fs231/en/
Malaria	Fact Sheet No. 94 http://www.who.int/mediacentre/factsheets/fs094/en/
Measles	Fact sheet N°286 March 2005 http://www.who.int/mediacentre/factsheets/fs286/en/
Plague	Fact Sheet No. 267 February 2005 http://www.who.int/mediacentre/factsheets/fs267/en/
Poliomyelitis	Fact Sheet No. 114 Revised April 2003 http://www.who.int/mediacentre/factsheets/fs114/en/
Rabies	Fact Sheet No. 99 Revised June 2001 http://www.who.int/mediacentre/factsheets/fs099/en/

Salmonella	Fact Sheet No. 139 April 2005 http://www.who.int/mediacentre/factsheets/fs139/en/index.html http://www.who.int/mediacentre/factsheets/fs139/en/index.html
Smallpox	Smallpox http://www.who.int/mediacentre/factsheets/smallpox/en/
Tuberculosis	Fact Sheet No. 104 Revised March 2005 http://www.who.int/mediacentre/factsheets/fs104/en/
Typhoid fever and Paratyphoid fever	Water related diseases http://www.who.int/water_sanitation_health/diseases/typhoid/en/
The World Health Organization	About WHO http://www.who.int/about/en/

GUIDELINES / PUBLICATIONS / REPORTS

Communicable diseases control in emergencies - A field manual. http://www.who.int/infectious-disease news/IDdocs/whocds200527/ whocds200527chapters/index.htm	WHO/CDS/2005.27 ISBN 92 4 154616 6
Protocol for the assessment of national communicable disease surveillance and response systems. Guidelines for assessment teams http://www.who.int/emc documents/surveillance/whocdscsrisr20012c. html	WHO/CDS/CSRIISR/2001.2 English only
Strengthening implementation of the Global Strategy for Dengue Fever/ Dengue Haemorrhagic Fever Prevention and Control http://www.who.int/csr/resources/publications/dengue/en/whocdsdenic 20001.pdf	WHO/CDS/(DEN)/IC/2000.1 English only
WHO report on global surveillance of epidemic-prone infectious diseases http://www.who.int/csr/resources/publications/surveillance/WHO_CDS_CS R_ISR_2000_1/en/	WHO/CDS/CSR/ISR/2000/1 English only
Guidelines for the collection of clinical specimens during field investigation of outbreaks http://www.who.int/emc-documents/surveillance/whocdscsredc2004c.	WHO/CDS/CSR/EDC/2000.4 English only
Hepatitis A http://www.who.int/emc-documents/hepatitis/whocdscsredc20007c.html	WHO/CDS/EDC/2000.7 English only
Guidelines for epidemic preparedness and response to measles outbreaks http://www.who.int/emc-documents/measles/whocdscsrisr991c.html	WHO/CDS/CSR/ISR/99/1 English only
Influenza pandemic preparedness plan. The role of WHO and guidelines for national and regional planning http://www.who.int/csr/resources/publications/influenza/WHO_CDS_CSR_ EDC_99_1/en/	WHO/CDS/CSR/EDC/99/1 English only
Plague manual: epidemiology, distribution, surveillance and control http://www.who.int/emc-documents/plague/whocdscsredc992c.html	WHO/CDS/CSR/EDC/99.2 English and French

Laboratory methods for the diagnosis of meningitis caused by *Neisseria meningitidis, Streptococcus pneumoniae,* and *Haemophilus influenzae* http://www.who.int/emc-documents/meningitis/whocdscsredc997c.html	WHO/CDS/CSR/EDC/99.7 English and French
Laboratory methods for the diagnosis of epidemic dysentery and cholera, 1999 http://www.cdc.gov/ncidod/dbmd/diseaseinfo/cholera/top.pdf	WHO/CDS/CSR/EDC//99.8 English and French
Control of epidemic meningococcal disease. WHO practical guidelines. 2nd ed. http://www.who.intlemc-documents/meningitis/whoemcbac983c.html	WHO/EMC/DIS/98.3
Guidelines for the surveillance and control of anthrax in human and animals. 3rd ed.	WHO/EMC/ZDI/98.6
Cholera and other epidemic diarrhoeal diseases control. Technical cards on environmental sanitation, 1997 http://www.who.int/csr/resources/publications/cholera/WHO_EMC_DIS_97_6/en/	WHO/EMC/DIS/97.6
Epidemic diarrhoeal disease preparedness and response. Training and practice, 1998 (Participant's manual) http://www.who.int/emc-documents/cholera/whoemcdis973c.html	WHO/EMC/97.3 Rev.1 English, French and Spanish
Epidemic diarrhoeal disease preparedness and response. Training and practice, 1998 (Facilitator's guide) http://www.who.int/emc-documents/cholera/whoemcdis974c.html	WHO/EMC/97.4 Rev.1 English, French and Spanish
Dengue haemorrhagic fever: diagnosis, treatment, prevention and control. 2nd ed. http://www.who.int/csr/resources/publications/dengue/en/itoviii.pdf	English only
Guidelines for the control of epidemics due to Shigella dysenteriae type 1 http://www.who.int/child-adolescent-health/Emergencies/Shigellosis_guidelines.pdf	Draft, 2005

VIDEOS

Protecting ourselves and our communities from cholera (41 min). http://www.who.int/emc/diseases/cholera/videos.html	2000 English and French

WEB SITES

WHO – http://www.who.int/
WHO/Cholera – http://www.who.int/topics/cholera/en/index.html
WHO Communicable Diseases and Surveillance – http://www.who.int/csr/en/
WHO Communicable Diseases Surveillance and Response –
http://www.who.int/csr/
WHO Infectious Diseases news, documents and Communicable disease
toolkits – http://www.who.int/infectious-disease-news/
WHO Roll Back Malaria partnership – http://www.rbm.who.int/
WHO Roll Back Malaria department – http://www.who.int/malaria and
http://www.who.int/malaria/complex emergencies
WHO/Stop TB – http://www.stoptb.org/
WHO/Water and Sanitation– http://www.who.int/water_sanitation_health/en/

16. List of publishers

The books and documents mentioned in this manual may be obtained from the following addresses. Some are available free of charge.

WHO Publications. Marketing and Dissemination, 20, avenue Appia, 1211 Geneva 27, Switzerland – Tel. +41 (0)22 791 2476, Fax: +41 (0)22 791 4857, E-mail: publications@who.int, Web site: http://www.who.int

Kumarian Press, Inc., 1294 Blue Hills Avenue, Bloomfield, CT 06002, USA Tel. +1 (800) 289 2664, Fax: +1 (860) 243 2867, E-mail: kpbooks@aol.com

Water, Engineering and Development Centre, Loughborough University, Leicestershire, LE11 3TU, England – Tel. +44 1509 222885, Fax: +441509 211079, E-mail: WEDC@lboro.ac.uk

Médecins Sans Frontières

International Office: Médecins Sans Frontières, 39 rue de la Tourelle, 1040 Brussels, Belgium – Tel: +32 2 2801881, Fax: +32 2 2800173

Belgium: Médecins Sans Frontières, Dupréstreet 94, 1090 Brussels Jette Tel. +32 2 474 7474, Fax: +32 2 474 7575

France: Médecins Sans Frontières, 8, rue Sabin, 75544 Paris Cedex 11 Tel. +33 1 40 212929, Fax: +33 1 48 066868

Luxembourg: Médecins Sans Frontières, 70, route de Luxembourg, 7240 Bĕreldange – Tel. +352 33 2515, Fax : +352 33 5133

Netherlands: Artsen Zonder Grenzen, Max Euweplein 40, Postbus 10014, 1001 EA Amsterdam – Tel. +31 20 5208700, Fax: +31 20 6205170

Spain: Médicos Sin Fronteras, Nou de la Rambla 26, 08001 Barcelona Tel. +34 9 3 3046100, Fax: +34 9 3 3046102

Switzerland: Médecins Sans Frontières, 78 rue de Lausanne, case postale 116, 1211 Geneva 6 – Tel. +41 22 849 8484, Fax: +41 22 849 8488

TALC (Teaching-aids At Low Cost), P.O. Box 49, St Albans, Hertfordhire AL1 5T, England – Tel. +44 1727 853869, Fax: +44 1727 846852, E-mail: talc@talcuk.org

UNHCR Headquarters, case postale 2500, 1211 Geneva Dépôt 2, Switzerland Tel. +41 (0)22 739 8111, Fax: +41 (0)22 739 7377

17. General references

Drugs and drug management

WHO model formulary. Geneva, World Health Organization, 2002.

Drugs used in parasitic diseases, 2nd ed. Geneva, World Health Organization, 1995.

Drugs used in sexually transmitted diseases and HIV infection. Geneva, World Health Organization, 1995.

Drugs used in skin diseases. Geneva, World Health Organization, 1997.

Management Sciences for Health, in collaboration with the World Health Organization. *Managing drug supply: the selection, procurement, distribution, and use of pharmaceuticals*, 2nd ed. Bloomfield, CT, Kumarian Press, 1997.

How to manage a health centre store. London, Appropriate Health Resources and Technologies Action Group, 1994.

Clinical guidelines, diagnostic and treatment manual. Paris, Médecins Sans Frontières, 2003.

Essential drugs. Paris, Médecins Sans Frontières, 2002.

The New Emergency Health Kit 98. Geneva, World Health Organization, 1998.

Materials

Emergency relief items: compendium of basic specifications. Vol. 2. Medical supplies and equipment, selected essential drugs, guidelines for drug donations. New York, United Nations Development Programme, 1996.

General medicine

Gregg MB. *Field epidemiology*. Oxford, Oxford University Press, 1996.

Lumley JSP et al. *Handbook of the medical care of catastrophes*. London, Royal Society of Medicine 1996.

Strickland GT. *Hunter's tropical medicine*, 7th ed. Philadelphia, WB Saunders Company, 1991.

Manson's tropical diseases. London, W.B. Saunders, 1996.

Eddleston M, Pierini S. *Oxford handbook of tropical medicine*. Oxford, Oxford University Press, 1999.

General : disasters and emergencies

Refugee health: an approach to emergency situations. Médecins Sans Frontières, 1997.

Handbook for emergencies 2nd edition. Geneva, Office of the United Nations High Commissioner for Refugees, 1999.

Perrin P. *Handbook on war and public health*. Geneva, International Committee of the Red Cross, 1996.

Brès PLJ. *Public health action in emergencies caused by epidemics*. Geneva, World Health Organization, 1986.

Community emergency preparedness: a manual for managers and policy-makers. Geneva, World health Organization, 1999.

Noji EK ed. *The public health consequences of disasters*. New York, Oxford University Press, 1997.

Rapid health assessment protocols for emergencies. Geneva, World Health Organization, 1999.